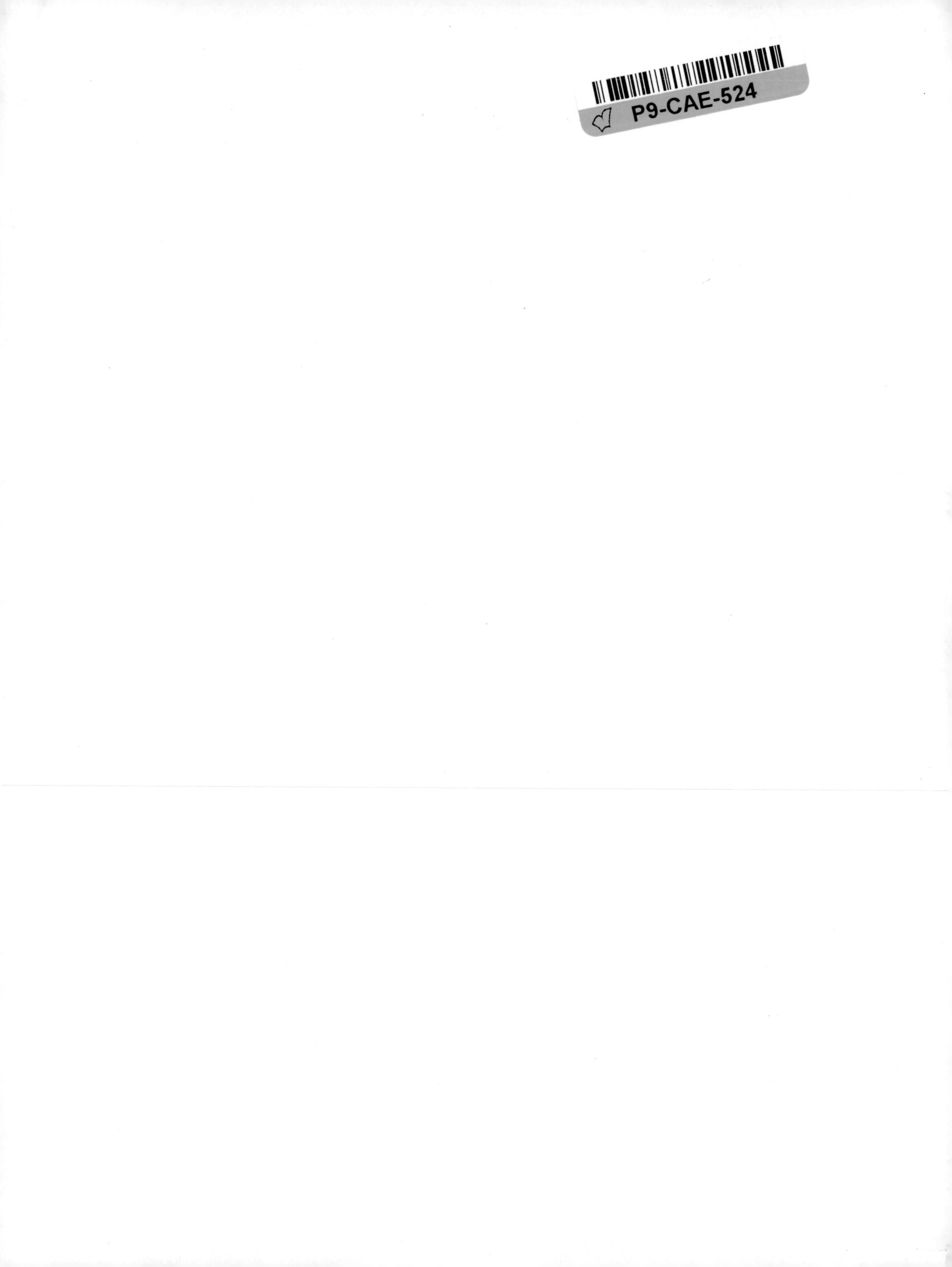
P9-CAE-524

Y's Way to PHYSICAL FITNESS

The Complete Guide to Fitness Testing and Instruction

Third Edition

Lawrence A. Golding, PhD
Clayton R. Myers, PhD
Wayne E. Sinning, PhD
Editors

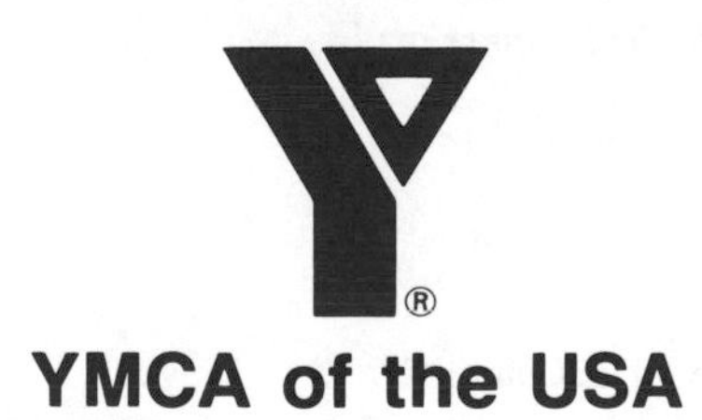

YMCA of the USA

Library of Congress Cataloging-in-Publication Data

Y's way to physical fitness.

Bibliography: p.
1. Physical fitness. 2. Physical fitness—Testing.
3. Exercise. I. Golding, Lawrence Arthur, 1926-
II. Myers, Clayton R. III. Sinning, Wayne E.
GV481.Y73 1989 613.7'1 88-27719
ISBN 0-87322-214-8

Published for the YMCA of the USA by Human Kinetics Publishers, Inc.

ISBN: 0-87322-214-8

Printed in the United States of America

10 9 8 7 6 5

Copies of this book may be purchased from the YMCA Program Store, P.O. Box 5076, Champaign, IL 61825-5076, 1-800-747-0089.

Contents

Preface

The YMCA has always emphasized physical fitness, but it was not until the mid-1960s that plans for a national YMCA physical fitness program emerged. At that time 50 experts in physical fitness, physiology, and sports medicine drafted a national physical fitness program for the Y. This proposal was presented at the First National YMCA Consultation on Physical Fitness held in Philadelphia in 1970. Two years later the first edition of *The Y's Way to Physical Fitness* was published. Certification of physical fitness specialists to administer The Y's Way to Physical Fitness program was instituted, and workshops were offered to prepare physical directors for this certification. The Y's Way to Physical Fitness represented a model YMCA program, one that originated at the grassroots level and involved many people.

As other national programs developed and The Y's Way to Physical Fitness program was used, the need to revise the program became evident. Norms were needed for women, and an advisory board was required to guide the new national programs in cardiac rehabilitation, weight reduction, back exercises, school health, and other areas. At the Second National YMCA Consultation on Cardiovascular Health held in Chicago in 1975, the decision was made to revise *The Y's Way to Physical Fitness*. In addition an advisory board was appointed, and a director of the National Cardiovascular Program was named.

In the next 10 years, hundreds of people were involved with the revision of *The Y's Way to Physical Fitness*. During this time the national program changed its name to the YMCA Health Enhancement Program. The national headquarters were moved from New York City to Chicago, and a new executive director of the YMCA of the USA and a new director of the Health Enhancement Program were also appointed. The revision of *The Y's Way to Physical Fitness* was completed and announced at the Third National Consultation on Health Enhancement held in Chicago in 1982.

Since that time, national YMCA programs have expanded, the population has become more fit, and new resources have become available. An excellent relationship between the YMCA and the American College of Sports Medicine (ACSM) allows YMCA physical fitness specialists to take ACSM certification and use the YMCA physical fitness test battery as the practical part of the ACSM certification. This led to the realization that another revision of *The Y's Way to Physical Fitness* needed to be undertaken.

This third edition has a number of changes and additions. First, it includes new norms for all tests based on results from approximately 20,000 participants. These norms are divided into six age groups for each sex. The percent body fat prediction for both men and women now is based on measurement of the same three or four skinfold sites. (Dr. Andrew Jackson and Dr. Michael Pollock were kind enough to develop these equations for us based on their original data.)

There also are new workload settings used for the bicycle ergometer testing and a change in the target heart rate range.

Added to this edition are new exercises (with illustrations), new topics in the question-and-answer section, supplementary information on principles of training, and updated listings of Y and outside program resources and requirements for Y professional training, including the new Physical Fitness Instructor certification. Appendices in the back include new, reproducible medical history, medical clearance, and informed consent forms, plus sample goal-setting contracts and volunteer job descriptions.

Although we, the editors, have collected and assembled this latest revision, it is to the hundreds of physical directors, workshop faculties, and students, as well as expert volunteers, that thanks must go. It is your help and input that made this revision possible.

Lawrence A. Golding, PhD
Clayton A. Myers, PhD
Wayne E. Sinning, PhD

Acknowledgments

The first edition of *The Y's Way to Physical Fitness* was compiled from the input of 50 individuals who are or were leaders in exercise physiology, sports medicine, and physical fitness.

Much of the work of this group is still contained in this third edition. Below is a list of the original research and writing team.

Donald C. Bingham
George Burger
L. Eugene Cantrall
James Chapel
Kenneth Cooper, MD
David L. Costill, PhD
Paul Couzelis, PhD
Thomas K. Cureton, PhD
William C. Day, PhD
Belvin Doane, PhD
David W. Dunsworth
Delmar Eggert
Charles Eising
Donald S. Fletcher
Rueben B. Frost, PhD
Emery Gay
John F. Gibbs
Warren Giese, PhD
John Gillingham
Lawrence A. Golding, PhD
M.F. Graham, MD
Russell Harris
Tom Harris
William L. Haskell, PhD
James Havlick
Gordon E. Hendrickson
Bernard Howes, DDS
Alfred K. Johnson
Jack J. Joseph, EdD
Robert Jurci
Ken Kendro
Russell Kisby
Robert L. McFarland, PhD
Roger Martin
Alexander Melleby
Clayton A. Myers, PhD
Francis J. O'Brien, DMD
Wes Ogle
Arne Olson, PhD
Stan Pedzick
Michael L. Pollock, PhD
Wayne Ray
Paul M. Ribisl, PhD
Robert Salisbury
Charles H. Shattuck, Jr.
Wayne Sinning, PhD
James Skinner, PhD
Jack H. Wilmore, PhD
Michael S. Yuhasz, PhD

The volunteers who served on the Health Enhancement Advisory Committee during the developmental period of the original book include the following:

E. Stanley Enlund
Samuel Fox III, MD
Gary A. Fry, MD
Lawrence A. Golding, PhD
Clayton R. Myers, PhD
Nanette K. Wenger, MD
Jack Wilmore, PhD

From the day the book was published, the editors realized that it would need to be not only revised but also rewritten to include the many women involved in YMCA programs and to add new national programs. With the help of many individuals and committees, the original book was revised. Virtually all physical directors who have ever attended certification workshops, and certainly the workshop faculties, provided ideas and suggestions for the revision—some formally, some informally, some written, some verbal. Some of the major contributors to the revised edition, especially those on formal committees, are listed below.

Nancy Albertson
Merve Bennett
Jeff Boone
Sam Brown
Joni Coe
Rich Escutia
Ron Fish
Herman Gohn
Glenn Gress
Andrew Jackson, PhD
Larry Johnson
John Joyce
Dave King
Phil Mallers
Dan Ochs
Pat Owens
Dennis Palmer
Sharon Plowman, PhD
Terrell K. Puffer
Jackie Puhl, PhD
Kent Rea
Ed Reeves
Pat Ryan
Jeff Sadowsky
Jim Scott
Jim Seidl
Neil Sol, PhD
Michael Thompson
Pat Thornton
Steve Totten
Dick Webster
William B. Zuti, PhD

Although the membership of the Health Enhancement Advisory Committee changed through the ensuing years, the committee encouraged the revision. Dr. William Zuti, who became the new director of the National Health Enhancement Program in 1980, helped to facilitate its completion. The members of the 1981 Health Enhancement Advisory Committee should be recognized for their contributions:

Samuel Fox III, MD
Lawrence A. Golding, PhD
William G. Hettler, MD
Charles A. Pinderhughes, MD
Michael L. Pollock, PhD
Jesse L. Steinfeld, MD
William B. Zuti, PhD

This latest edition is not a revision in the strictest sense; instead, it is an updating and streamlining. The major revision is in the new norms, which now reflect six age categories for each sex. These norms are the most extensive on the adult population in the United States. A special thank you to Anne Lindsay, who did most of the work in collecting raw data for the new norms, and to Kirk Golding, who did the computer programming. Anne is a former YMCA physical director who did her graduate work in exercise physiology at the University of Nevada at Las Vegas. Kirk Golding helped Cardinal Health Systems develop the original software for the Y's Way to Physical Fitness program.

In addition to the new norms, the body-composition prediction formulas used for determining percent body fat and target weight have been made uniform for both men and women. Each uses the same three or four skinfold measurement sites.

Four hundred questionnaires were sent to YMCA physical directors, and 150 were returned, giving input on needed changes in the revision. In addition, in

1986 a committee was formed comprised of Physical Fitness Specialist's Workshop directors and their physiology consultants. This group added to the present revision. The members of this group are the following:

George Babish
Tom Burke, EdD
Lawrence A. Golding, PhD
Mike Heilbronn
Prescott Johnson, PhD
Dick Jones
Stephen Kaye
Alice Kazanowski, PhD
Cliff Lothery
Powell McClellan, PhD
Dan Ochs
Gary Pechar, PhD
Steve Siconolfi, PhD
Wayne Sinning, PhD
Pat Thornton
John Usmial
Anthony Whitney, PhD

There are numerous individuals who gave valuable input and who unfortunately are not listed. *Y's Way to Physical Fitness* represents a true YMCA grass-roots program. It was conceived, developed, and revised by the users, that is, the leaders who administer it daily. For both revisions we have returned to the "trenches" to get input. This program is yours.

Lawrence A. Golding, PhD
Clayton A. Myers, PhD
Wayne E. Sinning, PhD

YMCA Health Enhancement Programs

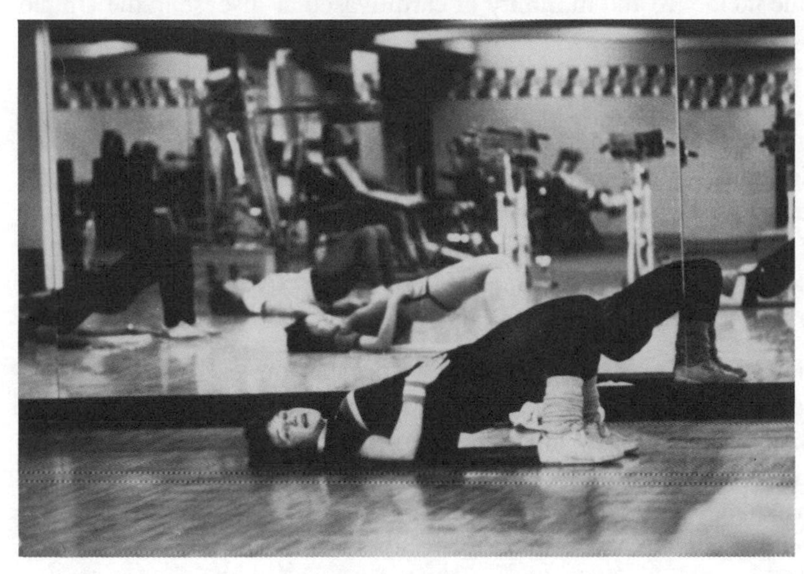

Chapter 1

The YMCA has promoted fitness and healthy lifestyles for over 125 years. Physical fitness programs have been a natural outgrowth of the Y's mission to develop mind, body, and spirit. Every YMCA program helps participants grow by

- encouraging them to set and work toward personal goals;
- providing opportunities to reflect on personal values and apply them to behavior;
- offering ways to improve personal and family relationships;
- helping them appreciate diversity in thought, culture, religion, and ethnic background;
- creating opportunities to become better leaders and supporters;
- developing specific skills to improve self-confidence and self-esteem; and
- providing ways to have fun.

The majority of Americans consider themselves to be generally healthy, but not enough of our national concern or resources are devoted to keeping them healthy. The ravages of heart attacks and other chronic diseases are being treated after the fact when preventing such tragedies would be vastly preferable and cheaper. By providing health enhancement programs designed to attack cardiovascular disease before it becomes crippling, the YMCA benefits an increasingly larger spectrum of the public by centralizing a wide range of cardiovascular health services. This plan, beginning with the education of youth and emphasizing health maintenance and disease prevention, is a natural extension of YMCA programs already in operation and provides for the addition of others to offer a wider range of services.

The health enhancement programs are designed to

- reduce the incidence and mortality of cardiovascular disease in the United States;
- help young people develop healthy values and lifestyles that may prevent cardiovascular disease;
- provide a medically sound exercise program for broad participation and to provide general information about health maintenance and enhancement;
- help identify those persons with increased risk of cardiovascular disease;
- conduct educational, motivational, and behavior-changing programs to stop smoking, control weight, and manage stress effectively; and
- develop and test new program models to serve special populations.

The idea is to offer programs that work to prevent the early development of coronary artery disease, to maintain health for those who are healthy, to promote early diagnosis of disease, and to provide rehabilitating therapy for those who have suffered heart attacks.

The health enhancement programs are built on decades of YMCA health and physical fitness leadership and are possible only because of great strides made by the YMCA in recent years. These accomplishments include standardization of a national program of physical fitness testing and proliferation of a national outreach physical fitness program.

The health enhancement programs have emerged at a critical time in the nation's history, when maximum use of resources and cooperative activity is being advocated, when there is discontent with the direction and cost of health care, when there is openness to health maintenance and disease prevention as a superior alternative to treatment of disease, and when the medical profession shows greater acceptance of allied health professions in meeting the health needs of Americans.

MAGNITUDE AND SCOPE OF CARDIOVASCULAR DISEASE

The problem of cardiovascular disease has been well documented, and the latest available data are published each year by the American Heart Association. Cardiovascular diseases are responsible for approximately 1 million deaths each year. Many millions more are afflicted but survive and are in need of special services. Major diseases of the cardiovascular system include high blood pressure, atherosclerosis, heart attack, stroke, congestive heart failure, rheumatic heart disease, and congenital defects.

High blood pressure is a silent and mysterious killer that may go undetected. In most cases the cause is unknown and there is no cure. Approximately half of those persons afflicted are not aware of the problem. If high blood pressure is not controlled, serious cardiovascular complications such as stroke, congestive heart failure, and kidney failure occur at an accelerated rate. At present, high blood pressure is the major disease suffered by America's black population and the most significant factor in their shorter life expectancies.

Atherosclerosis is a slow, progressive disease that often begins in childhood and sets the stage for heart attack and stroke. Autopsies of young servicemen during the Korean conflict revealed that the atherosclerotic process had often reached advanced stages, but early identification and modification of risk factors can retard its development. Poor eating patterns and excessive consumption of saturated fats and cholesterol point to the need for preventive activities to take place early in life.

Cardiovascular disease is the nation's number one killer, claiming more lives than all other causes of death. According to the American Heart Association's statistics, annual deaths average over 1 million. Approximately 4 million additional Americans have a history of heart attack and/or angina pectoris (heart pain resulting from inadequate blood flow to the heart muscle).

THE REDUCTION OF HEART ATTACK AND STROKE

The control of heart attacks is a major challenge for all persons and organizations interested in the nation's health. Increased screening activities and risk-factor education programs will help to identify those at risk and encourage early treatment. Extensive clinical and statistical studies of medical histories, physical conditions, and lifestyles have identified the major factors contributing to an increased risk of heart attack and stroke. These factors include heredity, sex, age, race, cigarette smoking, high blood pressure, elevated blood cholesterol, diabetes, obesity, electrocardiogram abnormalities, stress, and lack of exercise.

Some risk factors such as heredity, sex, race, and age cannot be changed; others such as elevated serum cholesterol, high blood pressure, electrocardiogram abnormalities, and diabetes can be altered by diet or medical therapy. General risk factors such as cigarette smoking, weight problems, lack of exercise, and psychological stress can be changed by the person at risk, and these are the major areas of emphasis in the YMCA programs.

Many studies show that people who lead sedentary lives have a higher risk of heart attack than those who get regular exercise. These findings provide the strongest rationale for YMCA involvement. Some individuals should exercise only with the advice of a physician. Exercise tests can be given to determine exercise tolerance and the reserve capability of the cardiovascular system, after which the appropriate kind and amount of exercise can be recommended.

The precise effect of correcting existing risk factors has yet to be determined, but the American Heart Association believes that risk-factor modification will reduce risk of heart attack and stroke and that the greatest improvements will probably result from simultaneously lowering all the appropriate factors. The best way to avert heart attack or stroke in later years appears to be by developing healthy lifestyles early in childhood. This approach, along with regular medical checkups and physical activity, is the foundation of the YMCA's health enhancement programs.

A COMMUNITY HEALTH PROBLEM

A new communitywide emphasis on early formation of health values, early diagnosis of cardiovascular disease, and greater availability of intervention programs is critically needed. However, a unified plan that offers this is not generally available to the public. Risk-factor screening and intervention programs should be added to the existing services of private physicians or health care clinics; but, because of the burden of acute illness placed on our health care systems, they often have been unable to emphasize preventive programs. This is a possible area where the YMCA can help.

YMCAs also are encouraged to work closely with medical organizations and American Heart Association chapters to develop exercise programs for the rehabilitation of cardiac patients. By working in tandem with such groups beginning in the planning stage, YMCAs can generate programs that will be satisfactory to all parties involved, including physicians and their patients. These programs can bring about psychological and physiological changes that improve patients' lives. The psychological changes include a feeling of well-being and a lower mental depression index; the physiological changes include a lower heart rate and a reduction of blood pressure, circulating catecholamines, and blood lipids. These programs also may help to define safe levels of activity for individual patients as well as to uncover abnormalities such as dysrhythmias that might otherwise remain undetected.

Rehabilitation programs are not always as available as necessary throughout the country. To aid in the effort to make rehabilitation programs accessible to all who need them, another purpose of the health enhancement programs is to maximize the utilization of existing facilities, personnel, and equipment to provide service on a broader scale.

PROGRAM OFFERINGS

The health enhancement programs presently available are the following:

- Y's Way to Physical Fitness
- The Y's Way to a Healthy Back
- Y's Way to Weight Management
- Y's Way to Stress Management
- YMCA Programs for New Families
- Y's Way to Strength Training
- Y's Way to Water Exercise

Y's Way to Physical Fitness

Y's Way to Physical Fitness was designed by a large and prominent group of physical educators, exercise physiologists, and physicians. It has become the standard YMCA physical fitness program because of its completeness and simplicity. Prior to beginning the program, participants must obtain medical clearance from a physician. Once enrolled, each participant should be given a fitness file prepared by a physical educator. The file should include the person's consent form and health and exercise history as well as records of performance on physical fitness tests. An exercise routine is established, and participants learn how to monitor their own workouts. They are instructed in nutrition, risk factors, caloric balance, and other health-related topics.

What Makes the Physical Fitness Program Special?

Physical fitness evaluation and the ensuing individual consultations provide special opportunities for lifestyle assessment and goal setting. The test battery provides baseline data so that improvement, which increases motivation, may be measured. Group exercise sessions become important social occasions, and the camaraderie leads to new friendships and support of personal efforts to reach fitness goals.

What Is a Typical Format?

After preliminary testing and screening, participants are assigned to group exercise classes conducted by qualified instructors. Some elements of exercise physiology are taught. Although most sessions are scheduled in late afternoon or early evening, some meet early in the morning or at noon.

What Materials Are Available?

Y's Way to Physical Fitness describes the organization, screening, and conditioning aspects of the program in detail. An inexpensive companion paperback, *Y's Way to Physical Fitness Leader's Guide*, contains a complete schedule for the Y Fitness Leader Certification Workshop. It includes discussions of basic principles of physiology and nutrition, overviews of fitness classes and leadership, and information on safety and liability concerns. *The Official YMCA Fitness Program* is the text for the leader's certification course.

What Training Is Available?

Certification is available for three levels: fitness leader, fitness instructor, and fitness specialist. A number of university-based workshops are conducted annually that offer a standardized curriculum and are administered through a national system. Thousands of physical fitness specialists have been trained to conduct this program in the past 5 years (see chapter 2 for detailed descriptions of training).

The Y's Way to a Healthy Back

The Y's Way to a Healthy Back is a special fitness program designed for persons who have experienced occasional or persistent backache or discomfort. It is preventive in nature and helps to relax and stretch tense and weakened muscles. Muscle tone and strength are gradually increased, thus warding off more serious and crippling back pain.

What Makes the Healthy Back Program Special?

Designed by a prominent physician and endorsed by a medical committee, the program can be easily learned and quickly organized. Minimal space and equipment are required. Long-term studies report that 80% of the participants improve the condition of their backs.

What Is a Typical Format?

In a typical back program 10 to 15 participants meet twice weekly for 6 weeks. Appropriate exercises are taught, and participants are encouraged to exercise daily at home. New exercises are added weekly, and recommendations for outside reading are made. Classes may start by using as little as 20 minutes and then gradually lengthen to 45 minutes.

What Materials Are Available?

The main text for the program is *The Y's Way to a Healthy Back*, which includes instructions for testing flexibility and strength in key muscle groups and outlines the 6-week program. The program exercises are described and illustrated. A videotape, *Say Goodbye to Back Pain*, also outlines the program and includes tests for discovering problem areas and tips on pain prevention.

What Training Is Available?

Workshops to certify instructors are conducted at regular intervals in each field. The 2-day course includes orientation, physiological and medical aspects of backache, test administration, exercise leadership, and marketing and other aspects of administration.

Y's Way to Weight Management

This program is more than just a diet class, as it takes a comprehensive approach to weight management that incorporates three equally important areas: eating behaviors, exercise habits, and food choices. It was developed by a registered dietitian and nutrition educator to help participants build healthy lifestyles that lead to permanent weight management.

What Makes the Weight Management Program Special?

As mentioned, emphasis is on permanent changes in behavior rather than the loss of a certain number of pounds or inches. The program is not only healthier for participants, but it helps them achieve control over their lives. It makes weight loss or maintenance a positive experience by turning healthy choices into a routine part of participants' lives and by utilizing group support and the continuing support of family and friends.

What Is a Typical Format?

Groups of 10 to 12 adults meet once a week for 10 weeks to learn about various weight management topics. Each session normally includes a review of the previous session; learning activities, which include a lecture, discussion, and written exercises; an assignment for the week, in which each participant establishes personal goals and plans; practice of a relaxation technique; and a wrap-up. Participants also are expected to keep a weekly record of their weight and a daily record of calories consumed.

What Materials Are Available?

Each participant should have a copy of the book *Y's Way to Weight Management*, which explains the major points of the program in easy-to-understand language and includes forms for various written exercises. For recording data about eating and exercise behavior, there is a *Y's Way to Weight Management Log*. The *Leader's Guide* provides the instructor with specific directions and lesson plans for leading sessions.

What Training Is Available?

Workshops to certify instructors are held regularly. Prerequisites are

- executive director approval,
- standing as a health professional,
- a sound basic knowledge of nutrition,
- good group-work and facilitation skills, and
- a positive, sincere, and caring attitude.

The course takes 19 1/2 hours, and, through a process of practice teaching and sharing, participants become familiar with the program content and improve their facilitation skills.

Y's Way to Stress Management

The unifying metaphor of this stress-reduction course is the idea of *management*. Just as an executive must learn and use certain skills to carry out business assignments, people must learn stress-reduction skills and utilize them on a regular basis. The skills include ways of coping with change, self-organizing, finding interpersonal support, keeping a positive outlook, building physical stamina, and developing a personal stress-management style. This program was developed by two specialists in creating stress-management and wellness programs.

What Makes the Stress Management Program Special?

Instead of offering generic answers to stress reduction, this program focuses on presenting skills and tailoring their use to each individual's situation. Information is presented from the viewpoint of a manager, providing the tools for each participant to set goals after seeing the overall picture, to determine priorities, to adapt, and to plan ahead. This program also allows participants to share information and solutions on a regular basis.

What Is a Typical Format?

Groups of 16 to 25 adults meet weekly for 8 weeks to learn stress-management skills. Every meeting includes the following: a group warm-up activity; short "chalk talks" that introduce three to five important points; written exercises that allow participants to relate information to their own needs; small-group sharing about personal approaches and problems; relaxation practice; and homework assignments.

What Materials Are Available?

Participants read the handbook for the course, *Kicking Your Stress Habits*, which guides them through the process of understanding stress, developing stress-management skills, and forming a personal management plan. Instructors read *Y's Way to Stress Management Leader's Guide*, which spells out how to organize and run stress-management classes and includes detailed lesson plans.

What Training Is Available?

Workshops to certify instructors are regularly presented. Prerequisites are

- executive director approval,
- standing as a health professional,
- a sound basic knowledge of stress factors,
- good group-work and facilitation skills, and
- a positive, sincere, and caring attitude.

The 16-1/2-hour course includes practice teaching and sharing of ideas so that participants can become familiar with the program content and sharpen their facilitation skills.

YMCA Programs for New Families

This group of three Y programs—You & Me, Baby; One, Two, Three Grow; and For Fathers Only—is designed to help pregnant women keep fit and to encourage parent-child bonding after birth. You & Me, Baby actually is a series of prenatal and postpartum exercise programs, one of which is an exercise class for both mothers and babies. One, Two, Three Grow is an activity program for parents and their toddlers to promote parent-child bonding and child development. For Fathers Only provides opportunities for fathers to interact with and learn more about their new babies.

What Makes Programs for New Families Special?

You & Me, Baby is a comprehensive program that allows women to begin exercising during their pregnancy and to continue afterward. It also includes optional water-exercise and strength-training components.

All three programs, besides improving fitness, enhance child-parent bonding and stimulate infant development. For Fathers Only is particularly good for involving fathers with their newborn children.

What Is a Typical Format?

You & Me, Baby is a series of programs for the mother and new baby that can be used in any combination desired. It includes the following programs: Prenatal Exercise, Prenatal/Postpartum Water Exercise, Postpartum Exercise, and Parent/Infant Exercise (for children from birth to 4 months or from 4 to 12 months). There also is a postpartum strength-training routine.

One, Two, Three Grow focuses on child-parent exercises, games, and activities that promote child development. Each session includes an attendance song and a song for the day, a warm-up, an exercise demonstration, exploration activities, a group activity, and a goodbye song. Classes may be organized for toddlers from 1 to 2 years old or from 2 to 3 years old and may run for 5 to 10 weeks. The program may also be offered as a class of aquatic exercises and water exploration, in which case each session consists of a greeting song, circle games, and a lesson in elementary water skills.

For Fathers Only is meant to help fathers enrich their relationships with their newborn to 1-year-old children. Six to eight pairs of fathers and babies meet for three 90-minute sessions over 3 weeks. (Some programs have run from 5 to 7 weeks.) Every session consists of a gathering time, a discussion, playtime, singing, information about parenting, and a closing.

What Materials Are Available?

The instructor's manual for all three programs is *YMCA Programs for New Families*. There is a participant's book for You & Me, Baby called *Exercises for Baby & Me*.

What Training Is Available?

Workshops to certify instructors are held on a regular basis. Prerequisites are

- executive director approval;
- certification as a Y's Way to Physical Fitness Leader;
- a sound basic knowledge of exercise physiology, correct exercise execution, and motor-skill development; and
- certification in cardiopulmonary resuscitation (CPR).

In addition, only males are eligible for certification in the For Fathers Only program. Participants have the option of becoming certified for one, two, or three of the programs. Course length runs between 22 1/2 hours for all three programs to 10 1/2 to 13 1/2 hours for a single program.

Y's Way to Strength Training

Strength training can be used in conjunction with cardiorespiratory exercise to provide a well-rounded fitness program. It can help prevent injuries by strengthening muscles in a balanced way. It also can improve appearance and is a fun and popular form of exercise.

What Makes the Strength Training Program Special?

Much of this program is designed for the average person, not for the avid bodybuilder. The suggested training workouts begin at a low level and gradually build to a more strenuous one. They are safe yet effective for developing muscle strength. Information is provided for setting up programs using Nautilus machines or Universal Gym machines and free weights.

What Is a Typical Format?

Strength-training programs are more individualized than are most programs. Class format is generally chosen by the instructor, although suggestions for developing programs are provided in instructor training.

What Materials Are Available?

Presently two books are available for this program: *Building Strength at the YMCA*, a participant's manual for beginning strength training, and *Instructor Guide for the Y's Way to Strength Training*, the training guide for the certification course.

What Training Is Available?

Courses to certify instructors are scheduled regularly. The prerequisites are

- executive director approval,
- certification as a Y's Way to Physical Fitness Leader,
- participation in a personal strength-training program,
- certification in CPR, and
- abstinence from drugs and all ergogenic aids, including steroids.

The course takes 18 1/2 hours: 12 in the classroom and 6 1/2 in practical experiences. Information is provided on organization, administration, and programming of strength-training facilities.

Y's Way to Water Exercise

Exercisers of all ages and at all levels of fitness can participate in this water exercise program. It is ideal for seniors and those who are overweight, pregnant, or physically disabled. It offers a safe aerobic workout, as the water's buoyancy prevents joint damage.

What Makes the Water Exercise Program Special?

This field-tested program includes exercises for each area of the body (lower, middle, and upper) as well as aerobic exercises. Instructors can choose the exercises that best suit their classes' needs. Three levels of exercise are described in the class plans: beginner, intermediate, and advanced.

What Is a Typical Format?

Classes usually meet three times a week for 8 weeks and consist of a warm-up, exercises for flexibility and muscular strength and endurance, aerobic exercise, and a cool-down. Games and circuit training are occasionally included to add variety and fun to classes.

What Materials Are Available?

Participants can read the book *Y's Way to Water Exercise*, which includes complete descriptions of all exercises with illustrations. The instructor may use the *Y's Way to Water Exercise Instructor's Guide*, which includes lesson plans for all three fitness levels, background information on exercise physiology, and recommended teaching methods.

What Training Is Available?

Training to certify instructors is available on a regular basis. Prerequisites for attending are

- executive director approval,
- certification in CPR,
- certification as a YMCA lifeguard,
- Basic Aquatic Leadership Course certification, and
- being age 17 or older.

The course runs for 8 hours, 6 of which are spent in the classroom and 2 in practical water experiences. To become certified the candidate must pass a teaching evaluation, demonstrate ability to plan and design an exercise class, and show an understanding of general fitness and proper exercise techniques.

A program that offers guidelines rather than a set program structure is the Y's Way to Better Aerobics. Instructors of aerobic exercise classes can use the text *Y's Way to Better Aerobics Leader's Guide* to design and lead their own programs successfully. Participants can learn more about aerobics and exercise from the book *Y's Way to Better Aerobics*.

The preceding programs and other Y offerings are included in the YMCA's plan for corporate health enhancement programs, *Health Enhancement for*

America's Work Force, a two-volume set. The *Program Guide* materials are designed to be used in conjunction with *Y's Way to Physical Fitness* testing and exercise formats. Directors developing corporate health enhancement programs will find both the *Health Enhancement for America's Work Force* publications, the *Program Guide* and the *Administrator's Guide*, to be helpful.

A LOOK TO THE FUTURE

The YMCA of the USA has identified the improvement of health and physical fitness as a major goal. Significant achievements have already been recorded by the YMCA in developing a nationwide pace-setting program with both preventive and therapeutic components. Prominent health leaders from several disciplines and representatives of key health organizations enthusiastically endorse our present activities and are urging the YMCA to move aggressively into health maintenance and wellness promotion with comprehensive enhancement programs. Present and future plans will be developed to do just that. For example, at this time the YMCA is forming a comprehensive youth fitness program to teach good health values and habits at an early age.

At the base of the YMCA of the USA's interest in expanding health enhancement programs and assuming an expanded leadership role in preventive health is the conviction that all individuals should have the opportunity to learn about health risks and how to reduce them. YMCA programs will be consistent with the idea of preventive health.

The first step is to give a healthy individual an understanding of his or her likelihood of developing illness through a knowledge of his or her personal risks and of the magnitude of those risks. This is done through educational classes and educational components in each fitness program. We then aid each person in reducing those personal risks. It is not enough to call attention to health hazards without offering alternatives. The YMCA provides opportunities for learning through personal consultation and education and for action through participation in fitness and recreational programs.

The Y is also in a prime position to develop healthy peer environments that may help foster behavioral changes toward improved health and lifestyles. Individuals, once alerted to their risks, may elect to choose appropriate actions to improve their well-being. This approach, coupled with the YMCA's continuing programs of exercise, education, and therapy, will enable us to broaden, almost without end, the horizons we seek to reach.

The preventive health programs of the YMCA, along with expanding private and governmental efforts, will help society reduce the cost of disease-oriented health care and help people better manage their personal health.

Planning and Organization

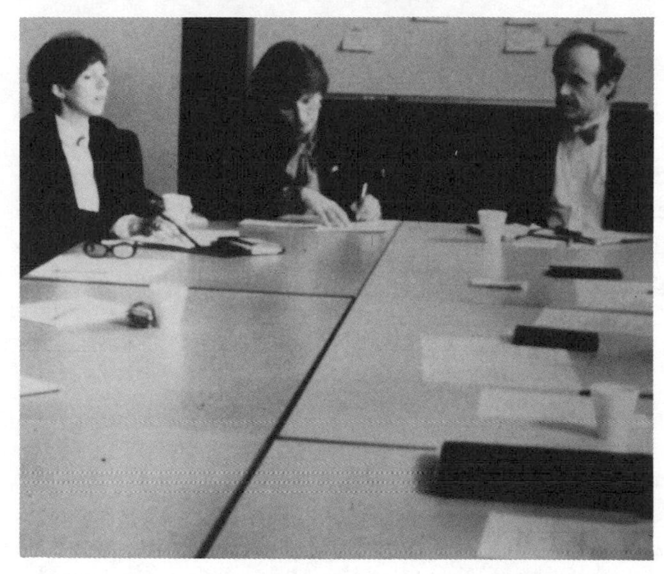

Chapter 2

This chapter provides guidelines for local YMCA volunteers and professionals for initiating or expanding physical fitness and health programming. The physical fitness programs briefly described in chapter 1 offer a vast reservoir of resources to facilitate local efforts.

Basic planning and organization are similar for all programs regardless of size or complexity. This process is presented in detail, though it is expected that some directors already use many of these sound practices. Just as portions of the national YMCA programs may be combined or modified to meet local needs, the planning process outlined here may be used selectively to fill gaps in local program administration. New program directors will benefit the most from this chapter by establishing these sound operating procedures early in their careers. Those who have additional experience or who work in YMCAs with already established programs will find this to be a good review.

PHYSICAL FITNESS AND HEALTH PROGRAM PLANNING

Many national YMCA programs are available and are described in detail in separate publications; however, supplemental local planning is essential to expanding existing programs or initiating new ones. When combined with the essential support of executives and the board of directors, these planning steps may very well be the crucial determinants of a successful program. It is the program director who usually supervises physical fitness and health program planning as described in this section.

Organize a Planning Committee

Early involvement of community health personnel is important for a YMCA that is planning or expanding its physical fitness and health programs. One of the better ways to secure this involvement and support is by organizing a *planning committee*. This representative group of professionals and leaders from organizations in the community—such as physicians, health educators, and corporate leaders—can bring valuable experience and depth to the planning process.

Review the Community Needs and Available Programs

In its first meetings the planning committee should discuss existing and projected programs related to physical fitness and health enhancement. Current successful programs that are priced fairly and well received by participants should be noted to avoid duplication. Committee members also may want to tour nearby facilities, participate in or observe classes, and obtain literature on other health enhancement programs.

The head of the planning committee then should discuss the national YMCA programs described in chapter 1 and circulate program materials for review. Gaps in community services will likely emerge, and the planning committee should be capable of assessing the YMCA's capability to respond.

Develop Objectives

When the information exchange and discussion process has been completed, the planning committee should begin to identify general and specific objectives such as the following:

General Objectives

- Provide opportunities for increased physical activity and health education.
- Provide leadership training in physical education and health sciences.
- Provide complete programs for all age groups based on currently accepted good practices.
- Recruit and train volunteers to assist in health promotion efforts.
- Serve as a physical fitness and health resource to community groups, business, and industry.

Specific Objectives

- Develop participants' cardiovascular function to delay degenerative changes typically associated with physical inactivity.
- Develop participants' muscular strength and endurance to meet the demands placed on the body through vocational and recreational activities.
- Develop participants' muscular flexibility around joints enough to assure

normal postural alignment, prevention of injury due to sudden strains, and full range of movement.

- Provide opportunities for relaxation and release of physical and mental tension.
- Develop an appreciation of the contribution of physical activity to general good health and a knowledge of the significance of different levels of activities, including sports, in fulfilling this role.
- Provide specific educational opportunities contributing to changed health behavior and improved lifestyles.

When objectives are clear, a more definitive description of needs and services is possible. Ultimately, this process leads to the development of policy statements and operating procedures. In developing such statements, planning committees should be aware of prevailing expert opinions of the potential contribution that increased physical activity can make to improving the quality of life. The new focus in health care is on prevention, in a personalized form, to reduce self-imposed degenerative diseases and costly chronic ailments. There is evidence that most serious illnesses, including the nation's leading cripplers, can be prevented by adopting healthier living habits and conditions. To this end, the YMCA can play a significant role by expanding its physical fitness and health efforts to include new elements of screening, problem identification, and education.

YMCA experiences are uniquely suited to this expanded role, which promotes personal responsibility for health, provides assistance in changing lifestyles, and contributes to high-level wellness. Boards and committees should consider these dimensions in establishing policies for local programs. The program director needs to keep the board of directors aware of the scope and quality of YMCA programs; in turn, the board members can help by providing additional program promotion and initial contacts within the community.

If the YMCA is to serve a community maximally, then all residents, students, and commuting employees must be considered potential consumers. More facilities may be required, and planners should be ready to schedule programs in non-YMCA facilities to fill the gap. Extension of YMCA programs into community facilities such as churches, recreation centers, meeting halls, and corporate centers offers the greatest potential for enrolling additional millions of people in health enhancement programs.

A systematic approach to identifying new participants should include a careful analysis of existing YMCA and community programs for each consumer group with different characteristics. The question "What exists and what is needed for which groups?" (e.g., seniors, preschoolers, adolescents) should be answered in detail.

Select Programs

When data have been compiled on existing and needed programs, the planning committee will be able to select programs that accurately meet community needs, consumer interests, and YMCA capabilities. The YMCA's health enhancement programs are unique and complete and are ideally suited for local YMCA implementation.

When target groups or special needs are identified by local planning committees, the probability is high that a YMCA program is already available to fill the need. If so, the initial work is greatly reduced. Parts of YMCA published programs may be used appropriately in combination with local elements. These published materials are attractive and well organized, and training and support systems are operating in each field for each program unit. Local YMCA identification with a national program strengthens the image of the YMCA and allows valuable data to be collected and compared. In addition, staff members develop skills and expertise that are transferable from one association to another.

Program selection may be influenced by the type of participant screening or medical clearance required or suggested. More important, programs should be selected on the basis of local capability to meet the program requirements. Some important criteria include the following:

- The importance or priority given to physical fitness evaluation
- The enthusiasm and support offered by volunteer boards, medical advisory committees, and chief executive officers
- The training and knowledge possessed by the individual who will direct the program
- The space available for testing and/or programming
- The amount of staff time that can be devoted to nurturing and administering the program
- The funds available to start the program and support it during its growth period

Identify Staff and Volunteer Leadership Requirements

YMCA physical fitness programs need the assistance of both paid staff and volunteers to directly lead program activities and develop policy as committee members.

Program Leadership

The number of personnel involved in a particular program will vary according to program size and complexity. A fully operative health enhancement center may be staffed by a director, plus one or more associate directors, fitness specialists, instructors, leaders, nurses, and physicians. Programs operating from smaller, off-site facilities might be staffed with one director and several part-time instructors. The major responsibilities for each staff position follow.

DIRECTOR: The director of a YMCA physical fitness program is officially responsible to committees and YMCA executives for all aspects of program management. This is usually a full-time YMCA professional position. The success of any program may depend on the dedication, enthusiasm, and drive of this person. The director should possess or seek to develop the following characteristics and skills:

- Warm personality coupled with group-dynamics skills
- Knowledge of the scientific basis of exercise, including exercise physiology
- Expertise in leading exercise classes
- Proficiency in testing and interpretation
- Ability to enlist, train, and supervise volunteer and staff personnel
- Skill in utilizing committee and community resources

- Competence in administration
- Ability to interpret and promote goals and programs
- Competence in CPR and current CPR certification

The director should be a college graduate with a physical education or exercise physiology major and a background in anatomy, kinesiology, physiology of exercise, and health education. He or she may have considerable fitness program experience and may have received specialized training at physical fitness institutes and workshops. Skills in group facilitation, counseling, and working with a board and committees are highly desirable.

The director should be able to plan, conduct, and administer a total physical fitness program, including leadership training and work with special consultants. He or she should know how to promote the program through mass media and should seek opportunities for personal interpretation of the program to everyone in the community.

ASSOCIATE/ASSISTANT DIRECTOR: The associate director should be able to manage with little supervision most responsibilities required of a director. Frequently, responsibilities are divided among the staff to utilize individual talents fully and accommodate personal work preferences. This is usually a full-time YMCA professional position.

PHYSICAL FITNESS SPECIALIST: A physical fitness specialist is a person who has received specialized training and who has demonstrated adequate knowledge of exercise physiology, physical fitness testing, test interpretation, and exercise principles. This can be a full- or part-time professional or volunteer. A specialist should be a competent group exercise leader and be capable of managing a fitness program. In particular, the specialist should possess skills in the following areas:

- Exercise-class planning and supervision
- Test supervision and administration
- Consultation with participants
- New program development
- Organization and administration
- Scheduling and supervision
- CPR

PHYSICAL FITNESS INSTRUCTOR: An instructor is, at the minimum, a talented, well-read, enthusiastic graduate of a YMCA fitness program who is willing to be trained to assist in the program. Training should include participation in a Fitness Leader's Certification Workshop. The instructor's usual functions are the following:

- Leading exercise classes
- Assisting with class organization, records, and special events
- Mixing with participants to offer encouragement and support and assisting those with special problems or limitations
- Assisting with test organization, administration, and clerical tasks
- Exhibiting competence in CPR

Instructors may be full- or part-time staff or volunteers.

NURSE OR OTHER HEALTH CARE PROFESSIONAL (HCP): Whether paid or volunteer, an HCP must have specialized undergraduate training in medical care. An HCP brings to the YMCA a solid knowledge of medical information, patient counseling, and emergency procedures. These skills complement and enrich YMCA physical education staffs. With the addition of programs for ''high-risk'' individuals, especially medically approved and supervised education and exercise programs for heart patients, nurses appear more frequently on YMCA staffs. Nurses should display the following skills and attitudes:

- Strong support of the role of exercise in improving total health
- Ability to interpret YMCA programs enthusiastically to community groups, physicians, and patients
- Cheerful acceptance of nonpatient duties as part of the YMCA team effort
- Ability to suggest ways to improve and expand YMCA programs in health promotion and lifestyle improvement
- Experience in a coronary care unit on a full-time basis
- Competent in CPR and advanced life support

PHYSICIAN: A physician is a person licensed to practice medicine in the state where he or she serves the local YMCA. Physicians commonly serve YMCAs in two ways: as volunteers serving on boards and committees and as paid medical directors of cardiac therapy programs. Specific services rendered include medical screening, test supervision, interpretation of electrocardiograms, and counseling. These services are often paid for on an hourly basis. Some YMCA directors prefer to pay physicians because of the implied increase in responsibility and accountability.

Whether paid or volunteer, the physician assisting in YMCA physical fitness and health programs should possess the following characteristics:

- Strong commitment to the YMCA program and an equally strong conviction that the Y has a unique contribution to make in the health field
- Current experience in the clinical practice of medicine
- Competence in reading electrocardiograms and in the supervision and interpretation of exercise stress tests
- Ability and enthusiasm for interpreting the YMCA program to community groups, medical societies, hospital staffs, and general practitioners.

Committee Leadership

Although volunteers can serve as program leaders, most volunteer leadership in YMCA physical fitness and health programs is through board and committee service. These groups, which often include highly qualified and generally recognized leaders in the field, help assure the quality and continuity of programs. Selection of appropriate committee members is usually based on the size, scope, and goals of programs.

Types of committees commonly selected are health and physical education committees and medical advisory committees. The boards set policy, and the committees take on an advisory role.

HEALTH AND PHYSICAL EDUCATION COMMITTEE: The Health and Physical Education Committee should sponsor the overall physical fitness program. Committee personnel should be totally familiar with the program and committed to its support. This committee acts as an advisory group for all physical education programs. It helps to determine the need for any additional committee structure in the area of physical fitness.

MEDICAL ADVISORY COMMITTEE: The Medical Advisory Committee is the crucial link between the YMCA and the medical community, especially when testing and evaluation is part of the program. The minimum requirement for a Medical Advisory Committee is a local practicing physician. Additional members may include other physicians, physical educators, psychologists and psychiatrists, nurses, physical therapists, registered dieticians, lawyers, and program representatives. Assure that community health organizations are associated with the fitness program through committee participation. Local affiliates of the American Heart Association, the American Lung Association, or the National Arthritis Foundation, the United Way, and local universities are a few examples.

When possible, representatives of the medical staffs of more than one hospital should be asked to serve. The medical director of a cardiac therapy program should be appointed by this committee. As medical director, that physician will be responsible for all medical services and education under general policies adopted by the committee.

A direct link from this committee to the Health and Physical Education Committee and the board of directors is advisable. This committee will carry out the following functions in accordance with YMCA of the USA guidelines:

- Review screening and medical requirements for participants.
- Set program standards.
- Endorse programs.
- Approve medical clearance and informed consent procedures.
- Review and approve medical aspects of all programs.
- Establish safe operating and adequate emergency procedures.
- Assist in program interpretation and promotion, especially to community groups, hospitals, and practicing physicians.

Medical advisory committees should consist of highly skilled specialists with potential to enrich the YMCA program. Because these individuals may not be familiar with the rich history of YMCA physical education or the broad scope of its current programs, a well-planned orientation procedure should be included as part of the meetings.

Identify Facilities and Equipment Requirements

The ideal situation exists when all aspects of a physical fitness program can be managed from a single location. Participants appreciate the one-stop convenience; administrators save time and money. A full-service facility would include a program director's office; space for registration, orientation, testing, equipment sales, lockers, and individual and group exercise; a jogging track; a swimming pool; showers; a testing laboratory; and meeting rooms. However, a program can be offered under less than ideal conditions, with proper modification of the exercise and education programs, when available space is found elsewhere in the community.

The program office should be large enough to serve the multiple purposes of administration, medical clearance, and participant interviewing and consultation. The testing area should be immediately adjacent to the office and connected with an emergency communications system. All doorways and passages should be large enough to accommodate a gurney and provide easy access to emergency medical units. The testing area should be at least 9 ft × 12 ft, with controlled temperature and humidity. Exercise areas should have a temperature range between 60 °F and 80 °F and humidity of less than 60%. An ideal fitness and medical evaluation center for large programs has been designed by Building and Furnishing Services of the YMCA of the USA. The multiple testing areas permit testing efficiency at minimal personnel costs.

Exercise and testing equipment will vary with the program selection, type of exercise, and budget. Specific recommendations are made by the physical director and executive director of each program.

Assure Adequate Insurance

Adequate insurance coverage for most fitness programs is provided in general liability coverage; however, such coverage should not be taken for granted and should be discussed early with the YMCA executive director and insurance advisors. When an additional amount of coverage or special coverage is required, there may be some delay. Although this could seriously interrupt schedules, no program should be operated until adequate coverage has been secured.

Attend to Start-Up Funding and Budgeting

Program directors should give as much attention to budget development as to program development. Failure to do so can result in early cancellation of a program that has solid growth potential over a longer period of time. Early detailing of start-up expenses and realistic projection of enrollments may indicate that outside start-up funding is required, in which case a proposal will have to be written that explains the program's purposes, financial requirements, and expected results. Responsibility for raising the funds must then be clearly assigned.

Program income is derived through membership and program fees and special agreements. Expenses include personnel salaries and fringe benefits, supplies, facility rental or upkeep, liability insurance, printing, staff training, equipment purchase, and maintenance. If program directors are inexperienced in such procedures, help should be secured from the local YMCA business manager or accountant. It may be helpful to collect several financial statements from other operating YMCA programs to avoid oversights or misjudgments. Ideally, a projected budget should be developed that covers a period of about 2 years.

Develop a Timetable

Achievement of objectives can be facilitated greatly by developing realistic time projections. When put into writing or graphic presentations, these target objectives clarify direction, organize staff, and provide some assurance that all contingencies have been considered.

Reaffirm Support

By the time the planning committee has completed its work, many original ideas and perhaps some priorities may have changed. At the very least, some financial projections will have been made that should be shared with the executive and board committees. At that time it is appropriate to reaffirm the organization's support to the necessary financing, staff, and facilities. Once this support is reaffirmed, the director and responsible committee are free to proceed.

ADMINISTRATION

The best administrative plan is one that has been written down and subjected to peer criticism. Once a plan has been completed to satisfaction, it becomes a valuable document that can assist in program interpretation, provide essential information for funding proposals, and serve as a blueprint for action.

An organizational plan must include effective means to organize resources, manage multiple levels of participants, utilize staff and volunteers effectively, promote participation, and operate the program smoothly.

Selection of Organization Pattern

If the physical fitness program consists of only a few programs and does not involve fitness testing or consulting, a minimal structure is acceptable. When professionally trained physical directors are not employed full time, allied health personnel, recruited to serve on a program committee, are helpful in formulating policy and guiding the program.

When full-time physical educators are employed and the program is more extensive, a committee devoted to physical education programs is recommended. Several members, including a practicing physician, should be recruited for their special interest and expertise in the fields of health and exercise.

As the fitness program expands to serve multiple groups and purposes, including fitness evaluation and risk-factor education, a medical advisory committee is appropriate. The director should be ready to seek the active support of physicians and other specialists in expanding testing and counseling activities.

A comprehensive organizational structure is required to manage large programs effectively. Several kinds of programs may be running concurrently, with exercise and testing assistance frequently being provided by trained volunteers. Testing is usually conducted at several levels and may include clinical as well as screening tests, requiring medical supervision.

Supervision of medical aspects of the program is the responsibility of the Medical Advisory Committee. The committee may be small, in some instances comprising only one or two physicians. One physician, actively practicing medicine in the community, should be designated medical director and have the responsibility of carrying out the established policies. Some of the issues commonly dealt with are the following:

- Review of protocols and endorsement of medical criteria for acceptance of new participants into new programs and continued participation in ongoing programs
- Establishment and periodic testing of emergency procedures, including supplies and equipment, for both testing and exercise sessions
- Prescription or approval of exercise programs for persons with special physical considerations

- Supervision and staffing of exercise testing
- Review of testing data and assistance in interpretation and counseling
- Promotion of program-related health education and risk education programs and assistance in staffing them

Where programs have reached this level of operation, the YMCA is likely to be operating jointly or cooperatively with one or more health-promoting organizations. Such collaboration is highly desirable and helps to minimize competitiveness and duplication of community services.

Volunteer Leadership Training

Probably the most important task facing any fitness program director is the maintenance of a consistent leadership philosophy and volunteer leadership-training program. This section further defines a leadership philosophy and presents an approach to training. To avoid repetition, we have assumed that the suggested training is cumulative or progressive. For example, the instructor is expected to know all that is suggested for the leader, and the director should master all skills and information required of the instructor.

The YMCA is considered to be a ''lay movement'' due to the extensive involvement of volunteers in all levels of activity and management. One characteristic of a competent staff director in the YMCA is the ability to attract and engage a wide variety of such volunteers. The importance of staff direction in recruiting leadership cannot be overemphasized. A functioning leadership development plan will result in a multiplication of programs and participants, provide a reserve of volunteers, give continuity to the programs, and enable the YMCA to offer quality programs at a reasonable cost to the participant.

Many opportunities for service and leadership exist in the physical fitness program, but recruiting and training volunteers is neither fast nor easy. It takes time and work, but it also pays great dividends in achieving association goals and personal satisfaction.

Potential volunteers should display the following characteristics:

- Firm belief in the contribution of physical fitness to a higher quality of life
- Regular participation in physical activity and a healthy lifestyle
- Sensitivity to the problems, needs, and limitations of others
- Enthusiasm, warmth, and cheerfulness

Leadership requirements will vary considerably, as fitness programs take different directions and vary in size. The most successful directors provide formal training for volunteer leaders and instructors, including a job description in writing. (For sample job descriptions, see Appendix A.)

A physical fitness ''leader'' will usually emerge from an operating program. He or she may be a participant who attends conditioning classes regularly and has derived health and social benefits as a result. This individual should exhibit enthusiasm, relate well to other group members, enjoy the exercise, look physically fit, and display leadership tendencies. Often this leader is identified by the director and groomed for leadership through a series of developmental assignments such as the following:

- Substituting on occasion when the instructor is absent
- Assisting in class administration

- Assisting class members who need special attention
- Assisting in the testing program
- Assisting in the conduct of special events or projects

Understanding the Scientific Basis for Physical Fitness

The volunteer instructor should understand the need for exercise as a part of a total health program. Most of the frequently asked questions related to exercise physiology are discussed in chapter 3. Specific areas in which instructors should be knowledgeable are the following:

- Principles of conditioning
- Effects of training
- Effects of body weight
- Signs of overexercise

Assisting in Planning and Administering Physical Fitness Tests

Skills in administering tests can be developed only through practice. A common mistake in many programs is that tests are given before the competency of the testers is proven. The director, instructors, and leaders should all participate in practice testing prior to actual use.

Instructors should be able to plan a testing clinic and assume the following duties:

- Promote the clinic and notify potential participants.
- Assemble and arrange equipment and calibrate bicycle ergometers and other apparatus.
- Prepare individual testing folders, organize recording forms, and compute fitness scores and profiles.
- Assign personnel on testing day.
- Direct traffic flow through the testing stations.
- Schedule individual interpretation sessions.
- Use audiovisual equipment effectively as necessary or appropriate.

Specific objectives of the physical fitness testing program are presented in chapter 4.

Training as Instructors

Many volunteers will function primarily as exercise-class instructors. All instructors should attend a Fitness Leader's Certification Workshop. In addition, they should read and be familiar with the material in chapters 3 and 5 of this text. The program director is responsible for seeing that volunteer instructors have read and understood this material. Finally, instructors must understand the procedures for physical fitness testing, record keeping, and first aid and emergencies, areas about which the instructor must be knowledgeable in order to conduct class.

Records and Reporting

Maintaining accurate records becomes increasingly important as programs expand. Early stages of record keeping may include only the number of sessions and the number of participants. As more personalized programs are added, more data will be gathered. This must be handled in a professional manner so that it is immediately available and yet kept confidential.

A system of record keeping should be developed and carefully maintained on group sessions, keeping track of dates, times, number of participants, instructor, supervisors, temperature, humidity, and lesson plans. Special incidents should also be noted, as well as how the situations were managed. Any special precautions, orientations, or instructions given to the group should be noted.

If testing is conducted, group summary sheets should be prepared. These summaries will be useful in evaluating class procedures, achievement of objectives, and cost-effectiveness. They will also be of value to program directors and researchers in modification of norms and program evaluations.

In personalized programs a folder should be maintained on each participant. This file, depending on the particular program, might include information such as the following:

- Registration data (e.g., date of enrollment, class dates)
- Consent and release forms
- Physician's approval or medical examination record
- Lifestyle assessment questionnaire
- Nutrition evaluation
- Statements relative to contraindications of exercise
- Coronary-risk profile
- Fitness-testing results and recommendations
- Attendance records and other physical activity records
- Notes on personal counseling sessions and referrals
- Progress chart (including resting heart rate, weight, laps run, sets and reps performed, target heart rate, and so on)

These group and individual records exist primarily to benefit the participant and the program manager. Additionally, they are a primary source of information for interpretation and promotion. Regular reports of significant personal involvement and group progress can help maintain internal and external enthusiasm for a program. Demonstrated results are also helpful when soliciting funds for expansion, equipment, or additional staff.

Promotion

The escalating public interest in physical fitness and health provides a constantly expanding reservoir of potential program participants. Few mass-media promotional techniques motivate these people to join the YMCA, so the fitness story must be delivered on a one-to-one or a small-group basis.

The best means of reaching new audiences is through well-developed personalized approaches to groups such as service clubs, industries, apartment dwellers, and church organizations. These presentations may be given by the program director, a skilled volunteer, or an invited authority. Another successful technique is to enlist the help of current participants. Satisfied participants can be valuable emissaries in a word-of-mouth campaign that reaches friends and business associates.

Information concerning all physical fitness and health programs outlining goals, exercise progression, and testing to be conducted should be sent to all physicians and health workers in the community. Asking for input and soliciting referrals from these people will keep the medical community aware of the programs and contribute to a positive attitude toward them. Give a free guest pass to potential referring agencies or agents and encourage them to use the facility or join the program.

Successful promotion of the physical fitness programs should begin with the YMCA staff and committees. Each individual should know about the programs and be able to discuss them with others.

- The executive director should be familiar with the goals of the program and be able to interpret them to boards, committees, and community groups to justify funding.
- The membership director should know the program details and costs and be able to explain them enthusiastically to potential participants. All staff who answer phones should be well acquainted with the program and should immediately refer any questions they are unable to answer to the appropriate staff member.
- The locker-room attendant should be friendly and helpful in giving directions, answering questions, supplying equipment, and keeping records.

Members of the YMCA board, the Medical Advisory Committee, and the Physical Education Committee should be asked to help in a second stage of promotion directed to the general public. This might include actions such as the following:

- Making announcements at service club and community meetings
- Helping to create and finance radio, billboard, and direct-mail advertising
- Helping to secure strategic locations for displays
- Making radio or television appearances (a considerable amount of free time is available to community service organizations)
- Helping to arrange demonstrations at fairs, sports events, and rallies
- Providing the staff person with a contact at a corporation

Some commonly accepted reasons why participants join and stay in well-run programs follow:

- Recommendation from a spouse, boss, neighbor, or friend
- Recommendation from a physician
- Desire to lose weight
- Desire to get in shape
- Fear of heart attack
- Enjoyment of social benefits
- Desire to be tested
- Acquaintance with someone who participates and enjoys it

These motivations, along with those that your committee and staff determine, should be the basis of organized promotion efforts. Research has shown that many people drop out of an organized activity or cease personal programs after only a few months. What can be done to maintain participation and enthusiasm? The following are some suggestions:

- Show results.
- Make class interesting.
- Vary exercise routines.

- Conduct incentive programs.
- Relate exercise to total health and efforts to quit smoking, lose weight, manage stress, and otherwise build a healthy lifestyle.
- Offer personal encouragement.
- Award attendance certificates, pins, and other symbols of achievement.
- Cite individuals as exemplary.
- Introduce fun activities and lifetime sports.
- Recognize achievement.
- Develop interest in leadership.
- Encourage bringing family, friends, associates.
- Abstract and circulate articles, research findings, and other pertinent information.
- Extend invitations to join the volunteer staff.
- Ask participants to set new goals periodically and put them in writing (see Appendix B).
- Send members to institutes and workshops as Y representatives.

Volunteer and paid instructors have a unique opportunity through close personal contact with participants to offer encouragement and promote continued attendance. Instructors can also be helpful by maintaining attractive bulletin boards and conducting public demonstrations. These activities are not automatic but require suggestion, cultivation, and encouragement from the director.

Interpretation of Physical Fitness Tests

Program directors may choose to interpret test results on an individual or a group basis or as individual follow-ups to group sessions. The choice usually depends on the type of program, the complexity of screening, the time available for testing, and convenience. The following should always be considered:

- Be aware of the psychological and medical implications that a participant may derive from the interpretation. Do not consciously or unconsciously make a medical diagnosis. If you are uncertain how to answer a participant's questions, do not cover up by giving information that may be incorrect but find the answer and relay it to the participant later.
- Consider all records when interpreting test results (e.g., medical histories, class attendance, personal observations).
- Give test results as soon after the test as possible. Undue delay reduces the impact.
- Make individual counseling available at times other than group sessions.

Knowledge that is basic to test interpretation can be gained by reading, studying, or learning specific published protocols and attending symposia and workshops. Skill in test interpretation can be gained through practice.

A cautious approach to physical reconditioning is advised. An important byproduct of the testing and exercise program is a changed and more active way of life; changing old behavior patterns and physically adjusting takes time.

Test results and their interpretation frequently are presented to participants individually in counseling sessions. Data for these counseling sessions are gathered from several sources. The individual file folder should contain information about health and exercise habits, medical history, and performance on physical fitness tests. Class records will supply attendance and work-capacity information. Personal observations are valuable in determining attitudes, behavior, and response to the conditioning program.

Counseling or test interpretation sessions work best when they are scheduled on a regular basis. Newcomers should receive counseling 4 to 6 weeks after the program is under way. Some repeaters may seek consultation, whereas others will feel it is unnecessary. The instructor should assume the initiative and set up special group sessions for test interpretation as needed. In addition to discussing how people are progressing, the instructor should be prepared to suggest exercise innovations to avoid monotony. With the wide variety of program options available at most YMCAs, there is no reason that a participant cannot find exercise options that are interesting. Instructors need to listen, ask questions, and use their imaginations.

As YMCA programs increase in variety and complexity, more contact with disabled people should be expected. Directors must be able to recognize program and personal limitations and confine their roles to guiding, consulting, and facilitating. YMCA programs are educational in nature and not usually staffed appropriately to help persons with pronounced physical, medical, or psychological problems. It is, however, helpful to have referral information available, including the names of professionals, public health agencies, and other specialized organizations. In making referrals it is essential to be sensitive to participant embarrassment, pain, or anger. An authoritative attitude should be avoided in favor of supportive questioning and suggesting. While offering support, directors should attempt to help the individual find solutions. Any referrals should be noted and follow-ups scheduled. The pattern of referrals and referral sources should be evaluated annually by the Medical Advisory Committee.

Emergency Procedures

Many participants are joining physical fitness classes for the first time and may be prone to accidents, both major and minor. In addition, although medical screening is suggested or required for all programs, some persons with borderline heart disease may go undetected. Procedures for giving prompt first aid and arranging for medical attention must be established in case a person has a heart attack while in YMCA facilities. A special emergency alert system should be planned that would immediately accomplish the following:

- Start CPR immediately.
- Contact medical assistance.
- Inform the director and front desk.

Fortunately, most emergencies and requests for first aid are for conditions far less serious than heart attack. However, every emergency should receive prompt attention under a detailed plan that includes the following provisions:

- Rendering first aid promptly
- Notifying the director
- Recording pertinent facts

Cooperation With Other Groups

Health and physical fitness activities in the United States have been expanding at a rapid rate. Numerous community groups and private entrepreneurs have recognized either the desirability or the profitability of programs, supplies, and services. All should be regarded as co-workers, and their offerings should be identified and evaluated when new or expanded efforts are contemplated.

Cooperative activity is both desirable and mandatory if the YMCA hopes to have full community cooperation. Planning among governmental, community, and corporate and private organizations contributes to a more equitable distribution of community resources and cost-effective services. YMCA directors can help bring this about by contacting local leaders, exchanging literature, establishing communication channels, and promoting referrals.

PROFESSIONAL LEADERSHIP AND TRAINING OPPORTUNITIES

Local YMCAs belong to the YMCA of the USA and support it through financial contributions and volunteer services. Monies received by the YMCA of the USA are divided among headquarters and the various field offices. The YMCA has developed several support systems for local YMCAs, including employment of full- and part-time specialists and program consultants. These staff leaders are the operational arms for the national health enhancement programs. To assist in this work, talented local directors are recruited to serve as field coordinators, cluster coordinators, and instructor trainers. Field coordinators are appointed by the field program consultants in conjunction with the national program directors. Their expertise and talents are utilized to promote national programs and provide training for others. After appropriate local clearance, appointments to cluster coordinator and instructor trainer positions are made by field coordinators and/or field program consultants in conjunction with national program directors.

Persons filling these positions should be the following:

- Certified YMCA fitness specialists
- Experienced in conducting successful programs
- Informed and current in exercise physiology, physical fitness testing, and health programs
- Interested in motivating and training others

The main responsibilities of the field coordinators and cluster coordinators are to coordinate program leadership training and to act as a communication link with local YMCAs. In addition, they are to do the following:

- Keep abreast of trends and developments in the fields of health and fitness, collect ideas and materials, and interpret and share the information.
- Plan, promote, and conduct fitness clinics and workshops.
- Seek opportunities to introduce physical fitness program ideas at conferences, meetings, and other events.

- Create publicity materials and opportunities to emphasize the need for physical fitness.
- Maintain liaison with, and promote membership and participation in, other groups working in health and physical fitness such as the American College of Sports Medicine; the American Alliance for Health, Physical Education, Recreation and Dance; the American Heart Association; the President's Council on Physical Fitness and Sports; and the Association for Fitness in Business.
- Relate the objectives of the physical fitness program to the broad social, personal, and Christian commitment of the YMCA.

Individuals interested in becoming a part of the national YMCA health enhancement programs are encouraged to contact field program consultants for program service. Field and national YMCA units conduct clinics and workshops. These events help local directors keep abreast of latest developments, meet other leaders engaged in similar activities, improve specific skills, and become more knowledgeable about physical fitness and health. Currently, three levels of training are conducted: Y's Way to Physical Fitness Leader, Y's Way to Physical Fitness Instructor, and Y's Way to Physical Fitness Specialist.

Physical Fitness Leader

This level of training is for volunteer and part-time class leaders. The following are prerequisites for enrollment in training:

- Executive director approval
- CPR certification
- A minimum of 10 hours of practical experience as a class participant or assistant instructor
- A healthy lifestyle
- Leadership qualities
- Basic knowledge of and interest in physical fitness principles

The workshop course is designed to give participants basic practical information on how to conduct an exercise class. It lasts 10 hours, of which 6 1/2 are classroom time and 3 1/2 practical demonstrations. Each workshop covers the following topics:

- YMCA history, philosophy, and programs
- The leader's responsibilities to teach and motivate participants and market the program
- The physiological aspects of exercise, such as heart rate and respiration
- Nutrition
- Safety and liability

Three demonstration classes are held, which are chosen from the following possibilities: starter, intermediate, or advanced fitness; choreographed exercise; senior fitness; strength training; and water exercise.

To obtain certification, participants must pass a written exam. This level of certification is a prerequisite for attending training for most other physical fitness programs (e.g., the strength training and the healthy back programs).

Physical Fitness Instructor

The second level of training is for experienced fitness or exercise-class leaders. The following are prerequisites for training:

- Executive director approval
- Certification as a Y's Way to Physical Fitness Leader
- A minimum of 15 hours and 2 months of experience as the primary class instructor since obtaining fitness leader certification
- CPR certification
- A healthy lifestyle
- Keen interest in physical fitness
- Leadership qualities
- An understanding of the role of fitness as a means to achieve the larger end of spiritual, mental, and physical development

The course lasts at least 11 hours, 2 of which are devoted to practical demonstrations. Topics covered include the following:

- YMCA history and philosophy
- Physiology
- Nutrition and weight management
- Body mechanics
- Y's Way to Physical Fitness testing and interpretation of results
- Special populations
- Medication and exercise
- Injury prevention and treatment
- Research updates

Certification requires completion of an evaluation form and a passing score on a written exam.

Physical Fitness Specialist

Training at this level is to prepare professional staff responsible for fitness programs. Prerequisites are the following:

- Executive director approval
- Certification as a Y's Way to Physical Fitness Instructor
- A minimum of 25 hours experience leading exercise classes
- CPR certification
- Practical experience in taking blood pressure
- Passing grade on a written pretest
- Completion of an informed consent form and medical release

It also is recommended that the candidate have a leadership role in health enhancement at the local YMCA and have earned a degree in physical education, exercise science, or health education. This course takes 45 hours, 22 of which are classroom time, 15 of which are practical experience, 4 of which are exercise sharing, and 4 of which are testing. The following topics are included:

- YMCA history, philosophy, and programs
- Physiology
- Kinesiology/applied anatomy
- Exercise principles and programming
- Anatomy and physiology of respiration and circulation
- Coronary risk factors
- Cardiac response to work
- Oxygen transportation
- Concepts of the measurement of oxygen uptake
- Metabolic equivalent (METs)
- Y's Way to Physical Fitness basic routine
- Y's Way to Physical Fitness testing and interpretation of results
- Diet, nutrition, weight control, and exercise
- Body composition and target weight
- Back home planning and organization

At least four exercise class sessions are held. Certification requires passing scores on both written and practical exams. In addition, certification is not awarded until the candidate has returned to his or her YMCA and completed 10 full Y's Way to Physical Fitness test batteries, sending the results to the appropriate office.

Participants who pass this course are eligible to take the American College of Sports Medicine Health/Fitness Instructor certification test without attending an ACSM workshop. The Y's Way to Physical Fitness testing procedures may be used for the practical portion of the test.

Further Training

Additional leadership training for all other YMCA programs is scheduled for training instructors. The field program consultant can provide information on these training events.

Occasionally, YMCA groups or individuals travel to other cities to participate in or observe another program in operation. This practice is highly desirable, as many new techniques and administrative shortcuts may be learned. Field and cluster coordinators can be helpful in identifying other YMCAs that have successfully implemented programs being considered.

Questions and Answers About Exercise Physiology

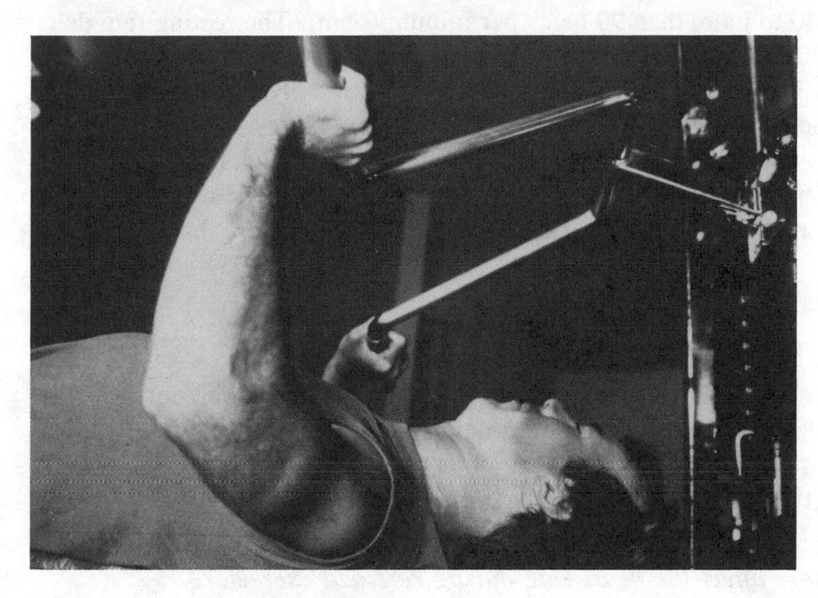

Chapter 3

This chapter is not written in the format of a text on exercise physiology. If it were, it would be a book in itself. Instead, the material is organized into pertinent subject areas that answer questions commonly posed by both fitness participants and physical fitness leaders.

Y's Way to Physical Fitness emphasizes programs for healthy men and women. The fitness leader, however, is frequently asked questions that pertain to problems more logically associated with cardiac therapy. Consequently, many relevant questions on cardiovascular function and diseases are included in this chapter. The fitness leader should be aware of physiological factors that indicate that it would be more appropriate for a person to exercise in a cardiac therapy program rather than a Y's Way to Physical Fitness program.

Reading and rereading this chapter should prepare leaders to answer correctly most of the questions they may encounter. A bibliography of additional information sources is presented in chapter 6 for those readers who seek more explicit information.

CIRCULATION AND EXERCISE

1. Is a low resting heart rate a good indicator of physical fitness?

Not really. There is great variation in resting heart rates; normal can range anywhere from 40 to more than 90 beats per minute (bpm). The resting rate does decrease with training, but this cannot be quantified relative to the amount of fitness. Slow heart rates, which are observed in extremely fit athletes such as swimmers and runners, do indicate cardiac efficiency. Occasionally a low heart rate will be associated with a physiological abnormality such as carotid sinus syndrome that is associated with arteriosclerosis. If it is desired to measure a person's resting heart rate, an average should be used to assure that a true base is obtained.

2. What is the maximum heart rate*?*

The maximum heart rate is the highest heart rate that one can elicit during exercise. Age is apparently the main determinant of maximum heart rate; as one grows older it gets lower. A rule of thumb is that 220 bpm minus age in years equals the estimated maximum heart rate.

3. What factors affect the heart rate during rest and exercise?

The heart rate can be affected by many environmental factors; temperature, humidity, emotional tension, time of day, time of last meal, smoking, drugs, and so on. If the heart rate is to be used in testing, steps must be taken to relieve emotional tension, maintain suitable environmental conditions, and assure that other factors are not operating.

It is especially important to know whether a person is taking medication if testing or using the heart rate to monitor exercise; this is especially true of drugs that are used to control high blood pressure. In such cases the heart rate is not a valid indicator of exercise stress.

4. What is the steady state *of the heart rate?*

When a person begins exercising, the heart rate at first increases rapidly and then continues to increase slowly for 3 to 5 minutes. It then levels off and remains constant during the remainder of the exercise. This is a steady state. If exercise is continued for a long period of time, a secondary rise may occur even if the work rate does not increase. The steady-state heart rate has value in evaluating fitness and measuring work intensity during exercise. Other physiological responses such as breathing and oxygen consumption will also reach a steady state in a similar fashion.

5. How is recovery heart rate *related to* exercise heart rate*?*

The heart rate begins to return to resting values at the cessation of exercise. The speed at which it returns depends primarily on the intensity of the exercise, providing there are no environmental factors affecting recovery. A quick recovery reflects a more efficient circulatory system.

The heart rate during the first 15 seconds following exercise is almost the same as the heart rate during exercise and can be used as an indicator of exercise intensity. The exercise rate is usually counted by having the exerciser find the pulse during the first 5 seconds following exercise, then count for 10 seconds starting the count on a beat, which is counted as "zero" and multiply by 6. It is usually easiest to give participants a target heart rate (see question 7) as a 10-second count. For example, if the target exercise heart rate is 140 bpm, the target 10-second count is 23 to 24 bpm.

6. How does the heart respond to different kinds of exercise?

Isometric or static exercise (i.e., exercise that works against a resistance that prevents movement) and heavy weightlifting cause reflex acceleration of the heart while developing a high resistance to blood flow and restricting venous return (the blood returned to the heart). As a result, there is an unusually high increase in blood pressure relative to heart rate and a possible reduction of the oxygen supply to the heart. Consequently, such exercises should be used with caution when working with adult groups who either have, or are susceptible to, coronary heart disease. Rhythmic isotonic or dynamic exercises will tend to increase the heart rate more than will isometric exercise while not adversely increasing the blood pressure. This is apparently due to the muscles' pumping action, which returns the blood to the heart, and to the lesser restriction to blood flow through the muscles. As the heart-rate increase during dynamic exercise occurs in response to the body's need for oxygen rather than as a nervous reflex, such exercise is more effective in improving cardiovascular efficiency than is weightlifting or isometric exercise.

7. How is heart rate related to inducing a training effect?

The heart rate can be used as an indicator of whether an acceptable exercise intensity has been reached, as it is highly correlated with energy expenditure. The workload during exercise should elicit a heart rate over 50% of the heart's maximum rate if it is to have a training effect. Normally, for safety reasons, an upper limit is given also, usually 90%, although athletes may work maximally.

The training heart-rate range or zone will, therefore, be 50% to 90% of the maximum rate. This may change slightly from group to group. The American College of Sports Medicine uses 65% to 90% as the training range, although different percentages are assigned to different levels of fitness: 50% to 70% for low fitness; 70% to 80% for average fitness; and 80% to 90% for high fitness. The YMCA is more cautious with the upper rate and uses 65% to 85% of the maximum as a desirable training heart-rate range.

The following example illustrates how target heart rate percentages are computed. To find the 70% target heart rate for a 40-year-old man, you would subtract his resting heart rate from his maximum heart rate. His resting heart rate, which in this example is 70, could be measured directly. His maximum heart rate probably would be estimated by subtracting his age from 220 ($220 - 40 = 180$). (This is safer than working someone to a maximum heart rate.) After determining 70% of the difference between the resting and the maximum heart rates ($.7 \times [180 - 70]$ or $.7 \times 110 = 77$), you would then add it to the resting heart rate ($70 + 77 = 147$). A heart rate of 147 would be 70% of this man's heart rate reserve.

8. What is an electrocardiogram*?*

An electrocardiogram is a recording of the electrical changes that accompany contraction of the heart. The machine used to make it is called an electrocardiograph. Both are abbreviated to the letters ECG (formerly EKG).

Changes in the electrical potentials of the cardiac muscle accompany contraction. Because the heart is bathed in an ionic fluid, these changes are transmitted away from the heart through the body fluids. Electrical sensors called electrodes placed on the body can pick up these changes and record them.

9. What are ECG leads*?*

These are the different patterns of electrode placement that are used to record the electrocardiogram. Sensing electrodes normally are placed on the right and left arms and the left leg. A "ground" electrode is placed on the right leg. This configuration yields six leads. There also are six precordial, chest, or V leads placed over the heart.

A 12-lead electrocardiogram is normally used. A standard procedure dictates the placement of the electrodes and their polarity so that all ECGs are comparable.

10. What does the ECG tell about heart function?

The ECG will detect changes that affect the normal electrical characteristics of the heart beat. These include irregular beats (rate and rhythm abnormalities), changes in cardiac muscle mass and position, tissue changes that occur with infarctions (heart attacks), and the effects of drugs and other chemicals. The interested reader should consult books on physiology and cardiology for detailed descriptions of these changes. The ECG cannot detect conditions that do not affect the electrical characteristics of the heart.

11. What is a stress ECG*?*

A stress ECG is taken while a person is exercising, usually on a bicycle ergometer or a treadmill. The test is usually progressive in the sense that the subject is exposed to higher and higher workloads until some predetermined end point is reached. Typically, the end point is voluntary cessation due to exhaustion. The test is always terminated when the ECG suggests impaired cardiac function or an unacceptable blood pressure response (see question 26). The stress ECG is sometimes referred to as the Maximum Stress Exercise Test (MSET) or the Graded Exercise Test (GXT). The stress ECG is a medical diagnostic test and must be given under the direct observation of a physician.

12. What is an abnormal stress-test result*?*

This is any test result that suggests the presence of coronary artery disease. Possible abnormal responses include the following, some of which are emergency situations that require the highest level of skill in medical resuscitation:

a. Exercise hypertension or exercise hypotension (see questions 26 and 27)
b. Chronotropic incompetence, or failure of the heart rate to rise with increasing workloads
c. Ventricular ischemia as indicated by the depression of the ST segment of the ECG tracing

d. Atrial arrhythmias including sinus arrhythmia (pacemaker), atrial fibrillation, and atrial flutter
e. Conduction defects

13. Why may having a stress ECG be important prior to beginning a training program?

A primary purpose of the stress ECG is to detect hidden heart disease. Between 8% and 14% of the normal population, who show no symptoms of heart disease, will show abnormalities when the heart is exposed to exercise stress. Such people may need a modified exercise program, or exercise may be contraindicated. The stress test also identifies the exercise intensity at which the individual shows abnormal cardiovascular response and maximum exercise tolerance. Both are important for individualizing exercise programs.

14. Who should have a stress ECG?

The final decision as to who will undergo stress ECG testing must be made by your medical advisory committee. Guidelines have been established by the American Heart Association (1972, 1975) and the American College of Sports Medicine (1986). (For additional information, see chapter 4, pp. 63-64.)

15. What are ectopic beats*?*

Ectopic beats are heartbeats arising from a foci (i.e., a spot in the heart wall) other than the sinoatrial node (SA Node). Normally the heart contraction starts with a change in the electrical charge in the pacemaker (sinoatrial node) and spreads over the heart. This is referred to as a depolarization wave. It first sweeps over the atria, causing them to contract. It then reaches the atrioventricular node, where it is transferred to the atrioventricular bundle and then to the ventricle muscle fibers, causing them to contract. Sometimes, especially after a myocardial infarction, areas in the ventricles become very irritable and depolarize prematurely, causing parts of the heart to contract out of sequence.

16. Can the individual detect ectopic beats?

Ectopic beats are apparent to the individual as ''skipped'' beats. Such beats might be noticed by the person while exercising. They can also be detected by taking a pulse. An occasional skipped beat is not cause for alarm; most people experience them occasionally. However, persistent skipped beats indicate that heart function should be evaluated by a physician.

17. In reference to stress testing, what is a false positive *test?*

Any irregularity of heart rhythm or indication of ischemia must be followed up by a medical evaluation. Sometimes medical examination will reveal a healthy heart even though there were abnormal responses during the test. Cardiovascular disease is a complex entity, and several symptoms must be evident to verify its presence. When stress ECG findings are not accompanied by other symptoms, it is called a false positive.

18. What is blood pressure*?*

Blood pressure is the force of the blood pushing against the walls of the arteries. The force is developed by the pumping action of the heart and two phases are identified: systolic and diastolic. *Systolic pressure* is the force developed when the heart contracts, whereas *diastolic pressure* is the force remaining in the arteries when the heart ends its relaxation phase and starts a new contraction. *Pulse pressure* is the difference between the two.

Blood pressure is measured with a device called a sphygmomanometer. Air is pumped into a cuff placed around the upper arm at approximately heart level. This closes the brachial artery, which runs along the inside of the arm. The air is then allowed to escape slowly from the cuff. The pressure in the cuff at the moment the force in the artery is great enough to push blood by the cuff is the systolic pressure. A distinctive sound that occurs with this event is detected from the artery by use of a stethoscope and tells the tester that systolic pressure has been reached. Pressure is further reduced in the cuff until the blood flows through even while the heart is relaxing. This point is identified by another distinctive sound change. Finally, the sound disappears. Highly accurate measurement of blood pressure during exercise can be attained only by sensitive instruments that require the insertion of sensors into the arteries.

19. What is meant by fourth-phase *and* fifth-phase *blood pressure measurement?*

As indicated in the answer to the previous question, there are distinctive sound changes that accompany pressure changes, and these can be picked up by the use of a stethoscope. Systolic pressure (first-phase pressure) is characterized by a loud "lub" sound. The second- and third-phase changes are very subtle and are of no concern here. The fourth phase is indicated by a distinguishable "lub-dub" sound, which some physiologists accept as the point of diastolic pressure. The fifth phase is signaled by the complete disappearance of sound, which other physiologists may accept as representing diastolic pressure. Hence, fourth- or fifth-phase pressures would be the pressures recorded at the respective sound changes.

20. How does blood pressure respond to different kinds of exercise?

Changes in blood pressure during exercise are somewhat dependent on the type of exercise. In moderate to strenuous rhythmic exercise (such as jogging), systolic pressure will increase, whereas diastolic pressure tends either to remain approximately the same as it was at rest or to decrease. In static exercise or dynamic exercise against a heavy resistance, both systolic and diastolic pressures tend to increase. Here, blood pressure increase relative to heart rate increase is much greater than it is in rhythmic exercise (see question 6).

21. What are acceptable values for blood pressure?

There are slightly different values given for acceptable blood pressure limits according to the source of information. The *YMCArdiac Therapy* manual defines *hypertension* (i.e., high blood pressure) as being greater than 150/90 and identifies four categories as follows:

- Uncontrolled hypertension—resting pressure consistently between 150 to 160 systolic and 90 to 100 diastolic
- Labile hypertension—resting pressure that varies, being sometimes above and sometimes below 150 systolic and/or 90 diastolic
- Controlled hypertension—resting pressure consistently less than 150/90 due to medication for hypertension

- Normal blood pressure—resting pressure consistently less than 150/90 *without medication* for hypertension

22. What is the cause of hypertension?

Hypertension is a symptom rather than a diagnosis. It can be caused by a number of factors, including kidney and endocrine malfunction. Approximately 95% of the cases are labeled as *essential hypertension*. This is a slowly developing condition that is apparently hereditary. Its onset is due to a number of interacting factors that are not easily identifiable. Treatment is a complex problem.

23. Will high blood pressure be reduced with improved physical fitness?

Studies on exercisers who had high blood pressure before starting a fitness program suggest that conditioning tends to lower abnormally high values. Exercise does not, in itself, bring blood pressure into acceptable limits. It can, however, help relieve some of the emotional stresses that are known to cause hypertension and can contribute to the reduction of body weight.

24. What concern should the physical fitness leader have about the blood pressure of someone entering a fitness program?

It is unsafe for a person with uncontrolled hypertension to exercise, as a stroke may occur during heavy exertion. Consequently, hypertension should be brought under control prior to starting a vigorous exercise program. This is the responsibility of the person's physician. Sometimes adjustment of the diet is adequate, but frequently medication is also necessary. The *YMCArdiac Therapy* manual recommends that a person not begin exercise if the resting blood pressure is higher than 160/100.

25. Are there special concerns that the fitness leader should have for someone who is known to have high blood pressure?

As a fitness leader you may be asked by the participant's physician to check the person's blood pressure before and/or after exercise. If you have concerns about an individual's blood pressure, refer the participant to his or her personal physician or consult with your own medical adviser. You should always know which of your class members are taking blood pressure medication. If you are using heart rate to monitor exercise intensity, remember that the heart-rate response will be suppressed in the medicated person and will not be a valid measure.

26. Is it possible to have normal blood pressure at rest but not during exercise?

Sometimes the blood pressure will be within acceptable limits at rest but will become unacceptably high during exercise. The *YMCArdiac Therapy* manual sets limits of 250 millimeters of mercury (mm Hg) systolic pressure and 130 mm Hg diastolic pressure during maximum exercise stress testing; the test is terminated if either is reached. Obviously, such values should not be reached in a routine exercise program. Exercise hypotension occurs when the systolic pressure fails to increase an acceptable amount with an increase in exercise intensity. This response indicates an impairment of cardiac function. Both exercise hypertension and exercise hypotension emphasize the need for a graded, maximum stress exercise test before entering a fitness program. Such a test is the only means we have of identifying these potentially dangerous problems.

27. Is low blood pressure ever a problem?

Some people may have very low blood pressure (hypotension) yet function normally. In such cases it is of no concern. Low blood pressure becomes a problem when blood flow to the brain, heart, and other vital organs becomes impaired. Chronic hypotension may be a symptom of cardiovascular or other diseases.

Blood pressure may fall briefly when we stand, causing syncope (sudden transient loss of consciousness), a condition referred to as *orthostatic*, or *postural*, *hypotension*. (True fainting is usually accompanied by some other emotional factor but is also accompanied by hypotension.) Postural hypotension may occur occasionally in anyone, especially when heat or some other factor places unusual demands on the cardiovascular system. Persons who experience frequent occurrences of postural hypotension should be referred to a physician.

28. What happens to blood flow during exercise?

During rest, the blood flow through the arteries and capillaries of the muscles is restricted because the smooth muscles in the walls of the arteries contract and hold the arteries closed. This process is called *vasoconstriction*. The resistance to blood flow due to this action is called *peripheral resistance*. When we exercise, these smooth muscles relax due to the effects of chemical changes in the fluids surrounding them—a process called *vasodilation*. In this manner, peripheral resistance is reduced, and more blood is provided to the exercising muscle.

The increased blood flow is accommodated by the massaging action of the muscles on the veins. The veins in the limbs have small valves inside them that permit the blood to move only toward the heart. Consequently, when the muscles contract and press against the veins, the blood is ''squeezed'' back to the heart with each contraction (see question 31).

29. What is ischemia*?*

Ischemia is a lack of blood flow to the tissues resulting in an inadequate oxygen supply. In the heart, this can interfere with the normal return to the resting electrical state and cause an abnormal ECG response. In the legs, this causes limping and periodic pain during walking, especially in the calves, a condition referred to as *intermittent claudication*.

30. What usually causes ischemia?

The usual cause of ischemic responses is atherosclerotic lesions, which are areas where cholesterol plaques are laid down with associated damage to the artery wall. Three places in the body develop most of the atherosclerotic lesions; the heart, where it causes coronary artery disease; the legs, where it causes arteriosclerosis obliterans; and the brain, where it causes cerebral arteriosclerosis. Arteriosclerosis obliterans causes intermittent claudication, whereas cerebral arteriosclerosis leads to vertigo, double vision, and other signs of cerebral impairment. It is also associated with stroke.

31. Reference is frequently made to the blood "pooling" in the legs. What does this mean?

During exercise the massaging action of the muscles accommodates the increased blood flow into the muscles by speeding its removal. If exercise is suddenly stopped, the metabolic factors that produced vasodilation are still present and the rate of blood flow into the muscles is still rapid. At the same time, the massaging action of the muscles is not present, so blood accumulates, or "pools," in the muscles until normal vasoconstriction is reestablished. Sometimes the amount of blood pooled is so great that there is not enough blood returned to the heart for it to maintain an effective pumping pressure. The brain and heart may be momentarily deprived of oxygen, which in turn may lead to fainting or may induce a heart attack with certain kinds of coronary disease.

32. How can one prevent this pooling?

The best way is to maintain the massaging action of the muscles against the veins. Do not suddenly stop after intensive exercise; instead, gradually slow the pace to allow the blood vessels to establish vasoconstriction gradually. An alternate way is to lie down and elevate the lower limbs.

33. What is the Valsalva maneuver*?*

During exercise against heavy resistance, when the breath is held, there is an increased pressure in the chest cavity. This pressure is transmitted through the thin walls of the large veins that return blood to the heart. The blood already in the veins is forced into the heart, which immediately pumps it out, causing a sudden increase in both systolic and diastolic blood pressure and in pulse rate. As the effort is continued, the pressure in the chest cavity prevents more blood from returning to the heart. Because there is very little blood to pump, the blood pressure and flow suddenly decrease again. This results in a decreased blood flow to the brain with resultant dizziness or fainting. The Valsalva effect can be prevented during these exercises by controlled inspiration and expiration, which periodically relieves the pressure buildup within the chest cavity and allows blood to return to the heart.

34. What are coronary risk factors*?*

Coronary risk factors are conditions that predispose a person to atherosclerosis and coronary heart disease. These include the following:

- Age—Incidence increases with age.
- Sex—Males are more frequently afflicted than are females, but after menopause the rate for women increases to almost that for men.
- Race—Black people tend to be at higher risk than white people. Black women tend to be afflicted at an earlier age than black men, white men, or white women.
- Heredity—Risk is greater in families in which close relatives have suffered heart attacks. This is especially true of heart attacks early in life.
- Hypertension—High blood pressure over 150 mm Hg systolic is another hereditary factor associated with heart attacks.

- Blood cholesterol—Any level of cholesterol over 250 milligrams (mg) per 100 milliliters (mL) of blood is considered dangerous.
- Obesity—Obesity is linked to a high incidence of coronary heart disease, probably because it is frequently accompanied by hyperlipidemia and hypercholesterolemia (high levels of blood fats) and by hypertension.
- Diabetes—Diabetics suffer a high rate of death due to coronary heart disease. This is especially significant among young women.
- Smoking—According to the American Heart Association, a person smoking more than one pack of cigarettes per day has nearly twice the risk of heart attack that the nonsmoker has.
- Behavior—Aggressive and/or high-drive individuals tend to have a higher incidence of coronary heart disease than have less stressed individuals.
- Inactivity—Lack of physical activity has been associated with a high incidence of coronary heart disease.

35. What are primary risk factors*?*

Cigarette smoking, hypertension, and hypercholesterolemia are considered primary risk factors. They are all factors that can be changed. Secondary risk factors are usually factors that cannot be changed, such as heredity, sex, and chronic health problems such as diabetes.

36. Can exercise reduce the probability of getting coronary disease?

The existing evidence on the beneficial effects of exercise on the prevention of heart attacks is largely retrospective, based not only on research but also on favorable experiences from physical fitness programs for normal, high-coronary-risk, and postcoronary people. Even though exercise has not been experimentally shown to affect the disease process directly, lack of exercise is still considered to be a coronary risk factor. Exercise has been shown to improve the physical capabilities of those who participate and to contribute to the reduction of body weight and body fats.

37. How does the high-coronary-risk or postcoronary participant benefit from exercise?

High-risk or postcoronary participants benefit from exercise much the same as healthy persons. They can perform more work without taxing the heart as much. Generally associated with this is more confidence and a sense of well-being. The participant develops the sense that he or she can still be a productive member of society and lead a normal life. However, a high-risk or postcoronary participant requires a special activity program and should not participate in the Y's Way to Physical Fitness program.

38. What is myocardial infarction (MI)*?*

Myocardial infarction is the death of heart muscle cells due to obstruction of an end artery. The size of the damaged area will determine whether the infarction is fatal or not. Myocardial infarctions are also more colloquially known as *heart attacks*.

39. How soon after a heart attack may the victim start exercising?

The *YMCArdiac Therapy* manual recommends that a new participant be at least 3 months beyond acute myocardial infarction, new onset of angina pectoris (see question 40), or an episode of unstable angina. For coronary bypass surgery patients, at least 2 months must have elapsed. In a hospital setting, postcoronary patients are sometimes exercised earlier than this on an individual basis with constant monitoring. The decision always should be made case by case with the help of the individual's physician.

40. What is angina*?*

Angina, or angina *pectoris*, is a sensation of squeezing pressure originating in the center of the chest. It is very diffuse, does not produce a sharp pain, and does not increase when a breath is taken. It often radiates, or spreads, from the chest into the jaws, neck, inner arms, or back. It may even appear in only one of these locations or spread from one of them to the central chest. Angina is usually triggered by physical exertion, acute emotional stress, eating, or exposure to cold air (the "Four Es").

41. Is it safe for angina victims to exercise?

Angina is one of the classic symptoms of coronary artery disease. Many sufferers (e.g., those who can control their angina with the drug nitroglycerin) exercise safely. It is important, however, that such people be properly tested before entering the program and that emergency equipment be available while they exercise. Angina victims belong in a cardiac therapy program rather than in a Y's Way to Physical Fitness program.

EXERCISE CAPACITY

42. What is maximum oxygen uptake*?*

Maximum oxygen uptake is the maximum amount of oxygen that can be transported to the body tissues from the lungs. (See chapter 4 for more about this topic.)

43. What is aerobic power*?*

The term *aerobic power* is used synonymously with maximum oxygen uptake, as the latter tells us the maximum rate at which we can utilize metabolic reactions requiring oxygen to produce energy. Such reactions are referred to as *aerobic*. Energy for physical activity may also be derived from *anaerobic* reactions, that is, reactions that do not require oxygen to provide energy. The amount of energy derived anaerobically is limited, so we must rely on aerobic reactions for prolonged activity. We expend approximately 5 kilocalories (Kcal) of energy for every liter of oxygen consumed. Aerobic exercises have been found to be more effective than anaerobic exercises in conditioning the cardiorespiratory system and in controlling weight.

44. Why is aerobic power used as a test of physical fitness, especially cardiovascular fitness?

The amount of oxygen that can be delivered to the tissue depends on the normal function of a chain of physiological events: (a) the ventilation (movement of air in and out) of the lungs; (b) the diffusion (movement) of oxygen from the lungs to the blood; (c) the blood picking up the oxygen, which depends in turn on the amount of hemoglobin the blood contains; (d) the heart pumping the blood; (e) the delivery of blood to the muscles by way of the arteries, arterioles, and capillaries; and (f) the ability of cells to use oxygen in the blood. The last step depends on the presence of microscopic structures called *mitochondria* within the cells and certain chemical substances called *enzymes*, which are necessary if the chemical reactions that use oxygen are to take place.

The oxygen-delivery chain is like any chain in that it is only as strong as its weakest link. Consequently, if there is a deficiency in any function such as the amount of blood hemoglobin, the distribution of the blood, or the pumping ability of the heart, the aerobic power will be reduced. Training improves many of these functions. For example, improved heart function, improved muscle capillarization, and an increase in cell mitochondria and enzymes are commonly accepted training effects. It is not uncommon to find improvements in aerobic power ranging from 15% to 20% with endurance-training programs such as those conducted in YMCAs.

It is also important to note that some people have naturally high maximum oxygen uptakes, apparently due to heredity. Many of them find success in competitive endurance activities. They may do well on physical fitness tests even though they are not in training at the time. They would be expected to improve with physical conditioning.

45. Does the maximum oxygen uptake tell us everything we need to know about a person's physical fitness status?

No. Strength, muscular endurance, flexibility, and body composition give important information in and of themselves. Participants still need to have medical examinations and clearance before going into the program. This measure can, however, give the program leader information about a participant's work tolerance and functional improvement due to exercise.

46. Does a high maximum oxygen uptake indicate a disease-free cardiovascular system?

No. A high maximum uptake suggests only good functional capacity. The person could have a high value and still be suffering from a cardiovascular problem that could be detected only by medical examination.

47. Is it practical to measure the maximum oxygen uptake in the YMCA?

For most programs the amount of equipment necessary, the technical skill required, and the danger of exercising older men and women to their maximum contraindicate the use of this test. Aerobic power can be estimated from submaximal tests. Such tests are recommended in chapter 4.

48. What is a physical working capacity (PWC) test*?*

The PWC test shows the amount of work a person can tolerate up to a specified level of physiological response. Usually the heart rate is used. For example, PWC 170 would indicate a work rate at which the heart rate would be 170 bpm. The PWC max would be the work rate that induces the maximum heart rate.

49. How is a PWC test given?

A subject is required to perform a series of more and more demanding bouts of exercise, usually on a treadmill or a bicycle ergometer. The heart rate is measured at each workload, and exercise is stopped when the target heart rate (about 160 bpm for a 30-year-old man) or some other criterion is reached. Lower target heart rates are used for older subjects (150 or 140 bpm). The YMCA's application of this concept is described in chapter 4.

50. How can the PWC test be used?

First, the PWC results can be used to evaluate physical fitness by comparing results to norms for age. The test also can be used to evaluate training effects, as after training a person will be able to do more work at a given submaximal heart rate.

In addition, the PWC can be used to determine acceptable exercises for a program participant. Assuming that a person reaches PWC 170 at a running speed of 8 mph, it can be expected that that person will not be overstressed by keeping the running speed below that level during the training program.

51. How are cardiorespiratory measures different between conditioned and unconditioned subjects, and what are maximum values for each of these groups?

Table 3-1 on page 46 shows values for unconditioned and conditioned groups on a number of cardiorespiratory measures.

RESPIRATION AND EXERCISE

52. What tests are there for pulmonary functioning, and what do they tell us about conditioning?

There are many tests of lung function, some of which include the following:

a. Vital capacity (VC)—the maximum amount of air that can be expired after a maximum inspiration
b. Timed forced vital capacity (FVC)—similar to VC, but the expiratory phase is completed as rapidly as possible
c. Forced expiratory volume in 1.0 second ($FEV_{1.0}$)—the volume of air expired during the first second of the FVC test
d. Percent $FEV_{1.0}$ of FVC ($FVC/FEV_{1.0} \times 100$)—the percent of the forced vital capacity that is expired during the first second of the FVC test

All these tests require the use of a spirometer to measure the air entering and leaving the lungs. There are many other tests available, but they are not commonly used in physical fitness testing.

The relationship between VC and physical fitness is indefinite. Obviously, it takes a certain lung volume to provide an adequate amount of oxygen during

Table 3-1 Cardiorespiratory Measures of Unconditioned and Conditioned Subjects

Measurement	Unconditioned Rest	Unconditioned Max	Conditioned Rest	Conditioned Max	Elite-endurance athlete Rest	Elite-endurance athlete Max
Heart rate (HR) bpm	72	190	60	190	40	200
Stroke volume (SV) mL	60	120	80	160	120	210
Cardiac output ($\dot{Q}$) L	5	22	5.5	30	5.5	40
Difference between O_2 content of arterial and venous blood [$(a - \bar{v})O_2$ difference] mL/100 mL	6	13	6	15	6	17
Oxygen uptake ($\dot{V}O_2$)						
$L \cdot min^{-1}$	.2	3.2	.2	4.5	.2	6
$mL \cdot kg^{-1} \cdot min^{-1}$	3.5	38	3.5	56	3.5	75
Respiration rate (f) breaths/min	14	40	12	50	10	60
Tidal volume (TV) L	.4	2.75	.5	3	.6	3.5
Minute volume ($\dot{V}_E$) $L \cdot min^{-1}$	5.6	110	6	135	6	193
Respiratory quotient (RQ) ratio	.82	1.2	.82	1.2	.82	1.2
Systolic blood pressure (SBP) mm Hg	135	210	130	205	115	215
Diastolic blood pressure (DBP) mm Hg	80	85	80	82	70	72

exercise. Some studies have shown an increase in VC with training, and others have not. Swimming has been shown to make the most improvement, whereas jogging has been shown to have very little effect.

Whereas VC is a measurement of lung volume, FVC and $FEV_{1.0}$ are indicators of the contractile force of the expiratory muscles. It is not uncommon for these measures to improve with training.

The percentage of the FVC expired at $FEV_{1.0}$ should be, as a rule of thumb, above 80%. Values below this suggest lack of thoracic mobility, excessive resistance to airflow in the lung passages, and ineffective removal of air from the lungs. It is not uncommon to find low values in asthmatics.

53. How is lung function related to performance capacity?

As the intensity of exercise increases (e.g., running faster), the demand for oxygen and air increases. There is a very close relationship between the amount of oxygen used by the body and the *pulmonary minute volume*, or the number of liters of air moved through the lungs per minute.

The maximum ventilation of the lungs improves with training. Untrained, middle-aged men may be able to ventilate only 40 to 80 liters (L) of air per minute. During hard exercise, a normal male college student will ventilate about 120 L/min, whereas exceptionally good distance runners may be able to breathe over 200 L/min for brief periods of time.

54. How frequently should one breathe while jogging?

The respiratory response is one of the most adequately controlled physiological mechanisms in the body; the less you interfere with it, the better. Let the body adjust as it will. When very poorly conditioned adults first come into the exercise program, they may become winded very easily due to their overall poor response to exercise. This is a sign of their inability to adjust to exercise rather than of their need to "learn how to breathe." As physical condition improves, the respiratory response will improve.

55. Are breathing exercises necessary?

Breathing exercises are of benefit to those suffering from chronic conditions such as emphysema or asthma. In addition, diaphragmatic breathing exercises and deep breathing can be used by healthy people to promote relaxation. Whether such exercises actually improve one's ability to respond to exercise is highly questionable, and long periods of breath holding should be avoided, especially after strenuous exercise.

ENERGY EXPENDITURE AND WEIGHT CONTROL

56. When does body weight become a concern?

Body weight becomes a concern when a person becomes excessively fat or thin. Both indicate a state of abnormal nutrition.

57. What is obesity*?*

A person is obese when he or she has excessive body fat. Here are definitions of some terms that may help you better understand obesity:

- Obesity—excessive amounts of body fat stored as a nutritional reserve
- Overweight—body weight greater than that allowed by some norm, usually based on age and height
- Underweight—body weight less than that allowed by some norm

58. Are obesity *and* overweight *synonymous?*

No. It is possible to be overweight and not obese. This situation is frequently found in large males who are physically well conditioned. It is also possible for someone to be of "normal" weight and still be obese if that person has excessively large amounts of fat.

59. What do the terms lean body mass *and* lean body weight *mean?*

The lean body mass (LBM) consists of all the body tissues exclusive of fat stored as a nutritional reserve. The lean body weight (LBW) is the weight of the lean body mass, usually expressed in kilograms or pounds. The *relative content*, or *percent fat*, is the percent of the total body weight that is fat.

60. What is a normal amount of fat?

Average relative fat values for males partly depend on age, but the new norms range from 16% to 25% of the total body weight. For females, the range is 23% to 30%. Males are considered to have too much body fat if they are over 30% fat and females if over 35% fat. Normal fat ranges would be better at 16% to 20% for men and 19% to 23% for women.

These values relate to people suffering from weight fluctuations typical of the general population. Excessive obesity is a special problem in and of itself, and people suffering from it present problems that cannot be readily handled in a typical YMCA physical fitness program.

61. What is the best way to measure body fat?

Age-height-weight tables traditionally have been used to assess body weight. However, more sophisticated techniques—such as body densitometry by way of underwater weighing or the use of anthropometric variables such as skinfold measures—are considered to be better. These are discussed in detail in chapter 4.

62. As so few calories are expended during exercise, is it worthwhile to consider exercise as a factor in weight control?

Weight gain and loss generally follow the laws of thermodynamics. A positive energy balance (caloric intake greater than caloric expenditure) results in weight gain. One pound of fat is equal to about 3,500 Kcal. Exercise programs such as those described in this manual require an expenditure of 400 to 500 Kcal per workout. This negative effect is cumulative and is equivalent to a pound of fat lost for every seven to nine workouts. On the other hand, eating a rich dessert once a day can easily result in an equivalent positive balance and an increase in weight. Energy equivalents of frequently pursued physical activities are shown in Appendix C.

Exercise does affect more than body weight. There are no advantageous changes in the cardiorespiratory and muscular systems when weight is lowered only by reducing the food intake. Usually it is best to control both food intake and exercise. Exercise as a factor in weight control is significant primarily for those who have only a mild obesity problem.

63. Sometimes exercises are rated according to METs. What is a MET*?*

A MET is the resting metabolic rate expressed in oxygen uptake or energy expenditure. It is assumed to be equal to 3.5 mL of oxygen per kilogram of body weight per minute, or .0175 Kcal of energy per kilogram per minute. If we say a physical activity has an equivalent of 6 METs, we mean that its energy demands are 6 times that of the resting state. The MET is very useful, as it accounts for differences in body weight without special computations. For example, assume that a 60-kg person and a 70-kg person were both exercising at 8 METs. The former would be consuming oxygen at a rate of 1.680 L/min and the latter at 1.960 L/min. Energy-expenditure rates would be 8.4 and

9.8 Kcal/min, respectively. The exercise intensity relative to the resting rate is the same even though the actual energy expenditures are different.

64. What are Atwater units*?*

The number of calories yielded by each of three components of food—carbohydrates, protein, and fat—varies slightly. Rounded off, the number of calories for each is the following:

Carbohydrate	1 g = 4 Kcal
Protein	1 g = 4 Kcal
Fat	1 g = 9 Kcal

These values are called *Atwater units* or *Atwater general factors*, named after the chemist Olin Atwater. The values are used widely by nutritionists to calculate the caloric content of food.

65. What about the use of vibrators to spot reduce or promote relaxation?

The energy cost of lying on a vibrating bench or chair is extremely low (.002 Kcal/min). Therefore, there will be no reduction in fat as a result of the exercise done. These devices are not effective in breaking up fat deposits or in changing the body composition in any other way. Some individuals may find them relaxing, but there is no scientific evidence that vibrators can spot reduce fat.

66. What about passive-resistance exercise machines?

Passive-resistance exercise machines have recently appeared on the market. These machines consist of a table or bench equipped with motors that move segments of the table or bench, in turn moving the body part resting on that segment, which supposedly exercises that part.

The concept behind these machines violates the basic physiological principles of exercise. Because the body part moved is not working against resistance, there is no increase in strength. Because there is no increase in heart rate, stroke volume, or cardiac output, no aerobic exercise is being done, so no calories are being expended. Although these machines may improve a joint's flexibility by moving it through a full range of motion, their value in improving muscle strength and endurance or cardiorespiratory fitness is negligible. They are of no value in weight reduction.

67. What about saunas, steam baths, and nonporous sweat suits for weight reduction? What about sauna belts, sweat jeans, and other devices designed to promote spot reducing?

These questions are related, and some basic considerations regarding dehydration need to be discussed prior to answering each. First, weight loss may be either temporary or permanent. If the loss is through dehydration, the loss of body water through sweating or through failure to replace water lost in other ways, it is temporary. Dehydration upsets the body's water balance, which the body regains as soon as it can by retaining any water later consumed. Therefore, an individual who dehydrates will rehydrate as soon as he or she starts eating or drinking again, and any weight that was lost will be regained. Weight loss by dehydration is sometimes referred to as *apparent* weight loss. Losing weight by dieting, that is, eating fewer calories than are expended, forces the body to get extra calories from stored food supplies. This negative calorie balance results in a weight loss that may be considered a real, more permanent weight loss.

Saunas and steam baths encourage sweating and hence a water loss that may cause a temporary weight reduction. However, because this is dehydration, the body will conserve water during the next few hours, and the weight lost will be regained. Weight lost in this way is no different from that lost by a football player who, on a hot day, may lose 5 to 7 lb during the game but who will regain the weight during the hours following the game.

Physicians are beginning to believe that saunas and steam baths may be detrimental to health. Heat stress is not tolerated well by most middle-aged people, and heat exposure can lead to heat exhaustion. The dangers of heat exposure are increased if an individual enters the baths after exercise, when the body is trying to reduce its temperature.

The same rationale applies to the use of the nonporous sweat suit. The nature of the material creates a hot environment for the body, causing sweating and thus a weight loss. This loss of water will be regained after eating and drinking.

Sauna belts, sweat jeans, and other such devices are supposed to promote spot reduction. These devices are made of nonporous materials that retain heat in a particular area of the body, thereby promoting localized sweating. Such local dehydration may cause temporary weight reduction, but there is no evidence that this will contribute to fat reduction. A Federal Trade Commission decision has restricted the advertising of these devices, as the evidence in support of the claims made was insufficient. The research literature reveals no evidence that spot reducing, either by heat or by exercise, is possible.

68. Many people claim that an increase in exercise leads to an increased appetite and thereby interferes with weight loss. Is this true?

Appetite is regulated to relate quite closely to energy expenditure over a wide range of exercise intensities. However, when a person exercises infrequently, the regulatory mechanism does not operate as effectively, leading to a caloric intake greater than the caloric expenditure, with the resulting weight gain.

69. Can one "change fat to muscle"?

No. When an untrained person participates in an exercise program, there may be a tendency for that person to lose body fat while increasing the amount of muscle tissue. Total body weight may remain the same. These are separate events that occur simultaneously.

70. What are "good" and "bad" cholesterol?

The body manufactures cholesterol because it is used in making bile salts that aid the digestion of fats. They also are necessary for brain and nerve functioning, and they form part of cell membranes. In the diet, cholesterol is found in animal foods. Triglycerides are another common type of fat in the body, generally found as stored fat. Cholesterol and triglycerides are important physiologically. These fats are transported by the blood and use protein as a vehicle of transportation. Such fat-protein units are called lipoproteins, and there are four major kinds: *high-density lipoproteins (HDL)*, *low-density lipoproteins (LDL)*, *very low density lipoproteins (VLDL)*, and *chylomicrons*. The most dense lipoprotein is HDL, which is about half protein. This is thought of as "good" cholesterol because HDL helps prevent heart disease. The lipoprotein with the most cholesterol is LDL, and LDL is considered the ''bad'' cholesterol because it is highly linked to coronary heart disease. Chylomicrons and VLDL are mainly triglycerides.

71. The terms hyperlipidemia, hyperlipoproteinemia, LDL, *and* HDL *are sometimes used in reference to the beneficial effects of exercise. What do the terms mean and what is the significance?*

Hyperlipidemia is an excess of fats (triglycerides and cholesterol) in the blood. Fats are carried in the blood on proteins, and when there is an excess of these proteins, we have *hyperlipoproteinemia*. These may be *LDLs* or *HDLs*. High LDL levels are associated with cardiovascular disease, whereas HDL levels have no pathological significance. Exercise is important, as it helps reduce high fat content in the blood. It has been found that regular exercisers tend to have a higher proportion of the HDL type relative to total blood lipoprotein.

72. How does one increase HDL and lower LDL?

Aerobic exercise, weight reduction, and cessation of smoking tend to increase HDL. Females tend to have more HDL cholesterol. One can lower LDL by reducing cholesterol and saturated fats and increasing polyunsaturated fats in the diet, maintaining a desirable weight, and increasing aerobic exercise.

73. What is the effect of exercise on cholesterol?

Intense exercise (300 to 500 Kcal in less than an hour) has been shown to reduce cholesterol in blood serum. A decrease in cholesterol occurs when there is a loss of weight accompanied by a loss of body fat.

74. What is the P/S ratio*?*

Saturated fats are found in animal meats and dairy products. Polyunsaturated fats are found in plant oils, and monounsaturated fats are found in particular plant substances such as olive oil, nuts, and avocados. The ratio of the polyunsaturated fats to saturated fats is called the *P/S ratio*. This ratio should be more than one.

75. What is the TC/HDL-C ratio*?*

The *TC/HDL-C ratio* is the ratio of total cholesterol to HDL cholesterol and has been shown to be predictive of coronary heart disease. To achieve a desirable TC/HDL-C ratio, the HDL level must be elevated and the LDL level lowered. Table 3-2 shows risk of coronary heart disease based on the TC/HDL-C ratio.

Table 3-2 Risk of Coronary Heart Disease Based on TC/HDL-C Ratio

	TC/HDL-C ratio	
Risk	Male	Female
Half the average	3.4	3.3
Average	5.0	4.4
Two times the average	9.5	7.0
Three times the average	24.0	24.0

THE UNIQUE PHYSIOLOGICAL RESPONSE OF FEMALES TO EXERCISE

76. Will exercise produce heavy muscles and "defeminize" women?

Research suggests that properly designed exercise programs improve rather than detract from femininity. Any tendency that a woman might have toward developing muscle bulk could be prevented by avoiding heavy resistance exercises (e.g., weightlifting) and emphasizing endurance-type activities.

77. Should a woman exercise during her menstrual period?

The ability to tolerate exercise at this time varies in different women, and each should exercise according to her own judgment. Many women have won Olympic medals while menstruating. The majority of women experience no change in performance during menstruation.

78. Can exercise relieve dysmenorrhea?

Dysmenorrhea (extremely painful menstrual periods) is often due to inadequate abdominal strength. Women who experience dysmenorrhea should not participate in activities that cause increased abdominal pressure on the pelvic floor during the menstrual period. This includes heavy lifting and hard vertical landings. At other times, participation in suitable exercises to strengthen the abdominal muscles and stretch the lateral trunk muscles should help improve the condition.

79. What are special problems women have with injuries during physical activity?

Injuries involving overstrain—such as contractures; inflammation of tendons, tendon sheaths, and bursae; and periosteal injuries—are more common in women than in men. The apparent problem lies in the lower ratio of strength to weight in the female. As a consequence, shocks and strains that would easily be tolerated by males may produce injury in females.

80. How does women's performance differ from men's in endurance activities?

Women tend to have a lower oxygen delivery system than men have. For example, on the average, women have less blood hemoglobin (the oxygen-carrying substance), a smaller blood volume, a lower stroke volume of the heart, and less muscle capillarization than men have. Women also tend to have a lower maximum oxygen intake per kilogram of body weight. This does not mean that women should not participate in endurance activities but rather that, on the average, their standards of performance cannot be the same as those for males.

81. Are training effects in women different from the training effects in men?

Although there may be differences between men and women in the rate at which they respond to training, the effects of training are essentially the same for both.

QUANTIFICATION OF EXERCISE

82. What is meant by the quantification *of exercise?*

The quantification of exercise involves putting exercise into measurable units that make it possible to select exercise that is appropriate for an individual's present health status and physical work capacity.

83. Are quantification of exercise *and* exercise prescription *the same?*

Both operate on the same principles in the sense that we are trying to individualize training programs. However, exercise prescription deals with special cases requiring medical supervision, such as those who have suffered coronary heart disease or are at risk of cardiac dysfunction due to multiple risk factors. Prescription must be supervised and approved by a physician. The same concepts can be used to assure that healthy adults who have been medically cleared will receive an exercise program adapted to their needs—something that good physical educators have done traditionally.

84. How is exercise quantified?

Exercise is usually quantified on the basis of its energy demands, either in calories or METs (see question 63).

85. What are the major factors to consider in planning conditioning programs?

Exercise programs to improve physical condition must take three factors into consideration: *intensity, frequency*, and *duration*. Intensity refers to the effort required to perform the work, frequency to the number of times the person works out each week, and duration to the time spent exercising. Research suggests that, for an optimal training effect, intensity of exercise be at approximately 70% of maximum capacity. Duration and frequency are interrelated; as frequency increases, duration decreases. However, research findings have suggested an absolute minimum frequency of three periods per week, with four periods per week being better. The total work done is a key factor. Therefore, a person should work longer during each session if the frequency is less. A workout equivalent to 250 Kcal per session is suggested for four times per week and 330 if three per week.

86. How can we monitor exercise intensity?

Exercise intensity is usually controlled by monitoring the heart rate (see questions 5 and 7). The heart rate during the first 15 seconds following exercise is nearly equal to the heart rate during exercise. Consequently, taking the pulse during this brief period gives an excellent representation of the exercise heart rate and thus the physiological stress.

87. What is perceived exertion*?*

Perceived exertion is how hard you feel you are working when you exercise. It has been shown in studies that if you feel you are working hard, you probably are. In fact, Dr. Gunnar Borg, a Swedish psychologist, has developed what he calls *perceived exertion ratings* based on the correlation between perceived exertion and heart rate, oxygen consumption, lactic acid levels, and other physiological responses. (See Table 3-3.)

Table 3-3 Perceived Exertion During Exercise

How does the exercise feel?	Rating[a]
	6
Very, very light	7
	8
Very light	9
	10
Fairly light	11
	12
Somewhat hard	13
	14
Hard	15
	16
Very hard	17
	18
Very, very hard	19
	20

Note. From G. Borg, "Perceived Exertion: A Note on History and Methods," *Medicine and Science in Sports,* **5**, No. 2, 90-93, © by American College of Sports Medicine, 1973. Reprinted by permission.

[a]The rating times 10 is approximately equal to the heart rate. For example, "Fairly light" = 11 × 10 = a heart rate of 110.

It is a good practice to take people's perceived exertion into account when deciding how to adjust exercise intensity, especially people who take drugs that affect the heart rate or who naturally have high heart rates during exercise. Ask them how hard they are working and look for the normal indicators of exertion (heavy breathing, sweating, flushed face) before deciding how to adjust their exercise intensity.

88. How is testing related to planning exercise programs?

Results from the PWC test give us an indication of a person's work tolerance. By comparing work tolerance to the energy requirements for physical activity, it is possible to select activities well within individual tolerances. The stress ECG becomes important when recommending training programs to participants who have a high risk of coronary complications or who have suffered myocardial infarctions. These people should not be in a regular program but rather in a cardiac rehabilitation program.

89. What factors other than test results must be considered?

Two factors of particular importance are age and physical condition at the start of the program. Older people cannot be expected to respond to training as rapidly as can youth. Programs for them should start at a lower intensity (e.g., 50% instead of 70% of maximum) and progress more slowly.

People in poor physical condition will experience a training effect at a lower work intensity than that needed by those in better condition. Walking is an activity that often will induce a training effect in previously sedentary people. Training programs for such people must be of low intensity to avoid overstressing their bodies and discouraging them by fatiguing them too much.

90. How much exercise can a previously sedentary person tolerate?

This depends on a number of important factors: the individual's age, health, whether the person smokes, how inactive he or she has been, and how long he or she has been inactive.

Almost anyone can start exercising at any time. However, the nature of the activity for the individual depends on the above factors. A 30-year-old man who has been sedentary for 10 years, does not smoke, is within normal weight limits, and is free of disease can probably do any program of exercise as long as he starts out slowly, exercises regularly, and progresses slowly but steadily. A 55-year-old man who has been sedentary for 35 years, smokes two packs of cigarettes per day, is overweight, and has some history of high blood pressure, high cholesterol, and diabetes probably should have a severely limited program of exercise involving walking and rhythmic flexibility exercises. The considerations will be determined by the person's medical exam, history, and physical fitness testing results. Common sense is the key guideline. Start at a low exercise intensity, progress slowly, and let the individual's responses dictate the nature of the exercise program.

ENVIRONMENT AND EXERCISE

91. What precautions should be taken when exercising in the heat?

First, wear a minimum of clothing. This allows sweat to evaporate more easily. Replace salt lost through sweating by adding more salt to food. Salt tablets are not advisable because of their high concentration of sodium.

Do not attempt to exercise too strenuously during warm days early in the hot-weather season, as the body must have time to make a heat adaptation. Although being physically fit makes heat easier to tolerate, fitness is not a substitute for heat adaptation. The only way to increase heat tolerance is to exercise regularly in the heat.

Even when heat adaptation has occurred, it is still important to be cautious. When heat and humidity are high, either cut back on exercise, increase activities such as swimming, or do not exercise at all. Exercise leaders should record the temperature and humidity in the gymnasium and outdoor exercise areas.

92. What precautions should be taken when exercising in the cold?

When exercising in the cold, whether it be running, skiing, or shoveling snow, warm up adequately by beginning to exercise gradually, especially if you are middle-aged or older. It may be desirable to warm up indoors in some instances. Do not exercise if this will force you to inhale excessive quantities of ice-cold air deeply.

Sudden cooling of the lower neck and chest can trigger reflexes that cause vasoconstriction in the heart. This reduces the heart's oxygen supply, leading to the onset of certain kinds of heart attacks. Try not to overdress so that you become overheated, but if you begin to feel warm, do not suddenly remove clothing and inadvertently expose these sensitive areas.

93. What about shoveling snow?

The same rules apply here as to exercise in the cold in general. Another precaution is in the size of the loads lifted. It is better to lift small loads more often than heavy loads less often. It may be wise to keep a small scoop available to assure that only light loads are lifted when working with heavy, wet snow. Lifting heavy scoops of snow is no different in its physiological effects from doing heavy resistance work in the gymnasium (see questions 6, 20, and 33). Generally the person who is physically fit and accustomed to strenuous activity does not need to be as concerned as the sedentary, unfit person does.

94. Are there any guidelines for judging the amount of exercise one should perform under hot or cold conditions?

When the weather is extreme, exercisers should use caution in how much they exert themselves. Table 3-4 and Table 3-5 provide guidelines for judging what level of workout to pursue.

Table 3-4 Heat and Humidity Chart

Relative humidity	Air temperature (F°) 70°	75°	80°	85°	90°	95°	100°	105°	110°	115°	120°
30%	67	73	78	84	90	96	104	113	123	135	148
40%	68	74	79	86	93	101	110	123	137	151	
50%	69	75	81	88	96	107	120	135	150		
60%	70	76	82	90	100	114	132	149			
70%	70	77	85	93	106	124	144				
80%	71	78	86	97	113	136					
90%	71	79	88	102	122						
100%	72	80	91	108							

☐ Risk of heat exhaustion ☐ Risk of heat stroke ☐ High risk of heat stroke

Note. Numbers within chart show equivalent temperatures. Shaded areas indicate when exertion may be dangerous. Reproduced with permission of *The Walking Magazine*, copyright © 1987, Raben Publishing Co., 711 Boylston St., Boston, MA 02116.

Table 3-5 Wind Chill Chart

Estimated wind speed (mph)	Air temperature (°F) 50	40	30	20	10	0	−10	−20	−30	−40
	Equivalent temperature (°F)									
Calm	50	40	30	20	10	0	−10	−20	−30	−40
5	48	37	27	16	6	−5	−15	−26	−36	−47
10	40	28	16	4	−9	−21	−33	−46	−58	−70
15	36	22	9	−5	−18	−36	−45	−58	−72	−85
20	32	18	4	−10	−25	−39	−53	−67	−82	−96
25	30	16	0	−15	−29	−44	−59	−74	−88	−104
30	28	13	−2	−18	−33	−48	−63	−79	−94	−109
35	27	11	−4	−20	−35	−49	−67	−83	−98	−113
40	26	10	−6	−21	−37	−53	−69	−85	−100	−116
Wind speeds over 40 mph have little additional effect	Little danger for properly clothed person				Increasing danger DANGER OF FREEZING EXPOSED FLESH			Great danger		

Temperatures assume dry conditions. The greater the moisture, the higher the temperature at which your skin may be in danger.

Note. Reproduced with permission of *The Walking Magazine*, copyright © 1987, Raben Publishing Co., 711 Boylston St., Boston, MA 02116.

95. What is the best time of day to exercise?

There is no time of day most suitable for exercising; this is best determined by each individual relative to his or her own daily schedule. However, at least 1 hour should elapse before exercising strenuously after a heavy meal. What is more important than the time of day is the regularity with which the person exercises each week.

96. What is the effect of air pollution on exercise?

Information is limited about how the exercising person reacts to air pollution. However, it is known that some people do have allergic reactions to dust or specific chemicals that produce bronchospasm (closing of the airways); this condition may be a severe problem in asthmatics. Carbon monoxide in the air reduces the oxygen transport capacity of the blood. This is compensated for by a higher exercise heart rate. Excessive ozone has also been found to cause small airway obstruction. Until we have more specific information available, it is best to use common sense and restrict exercise when air pollution is high and seems to add physiological stress during physical exertion.

97. Is it dangerous to exercise at high altitude?

The air is thinner at higher altitudes; that is, there are fewer oxygen molecules per liter of air. At some point the amount of oxygen carried by the blood is reduced, a condition called *hypoxia*. Under hypoxic conditions, work capacity is reduced, and any given task utilizes a greater proportion of reserves. At extremely high altitudes, such as those attained by mountain climbers, other physiological problems such as disturbance of the acid-base balance may occur.

For the healthy person, the effects of high altitude are annoying but not dangerous. For the person with coronary heart disease, however, it is considered prudent to avoid exercise at high altitudes, as the heart muscle's oxygen supply is already compromised. The *YMCArdiac Therapy* manual suggests that such people exercise up to altitudes of only 6,000 ft, or at the same air pressure level at which airplanes are pressurized.

ADDITIONAL QUESTIONS

98. What causes the muscle soreness so common among new program participants?

There are two types of pain resulting from overexertion. One is pain during and immediately after exercise, which is probably due to waste products formed during exercise that are left in the fluids that surround the cells. The other is a localized, delayed soreness that appears in 24 to 48 hours. The second type can become chronic and serve as a deterrent to further exercise. Whether it is due to small muscle tears or to small localized contractures of muscles is not known. Temporary soreness is a common phenomenon when doing a new exercise or increasing intensity and should not be a deterrent to continued participation in the program. Chronic soreness requires medical evaluation.

99. Can muscle soreness be prevented?

A conservative approach to exercise is the key to preventing soreness. Use a proper warm-up; gradually increase the workload during exercise; stay within the exercise intensity tolerance level of your group; slowly increase the amount of exercise performed from workout to workout; do not overdo a given exercise; gradually decrease exercise intensity at the end of the workout; and avoid bouncing when doing stretching exercises so as not to force the joints past the limits of their ranges of motion. Static stretching has been found to be effective in helping to prevent and relieve muscle soreness.

100. Is there any danger of collapse while showering after exercising?

Hot showers after exercise have been associated with arrhythmias and myocardial infarctions in people who have a tendency to such conditions. Apparently the vasodilation associated with exercise may be increased after a hot shower, leading to hypotension and syncope and producing the irregular beats or infarction. This should not be a problem in the typical Y's Way to Physical Fitness program. Participants should, however, be encouraged to take short showers at moderate temperatures. The locker room should be supervised until the last person leaves. Anyone experiencing chest pain during or after showering should be rushed to a hospital without taking time to dress (see question 40 on angina).

101. Lactic acid is mentioned frequently relative to exercise physiology. What is it?

Lactic acid is a chemical substance formed when the body is not meeting the requirements of the cells for oxygen (anaerobic exercise). It is important because its formation provides a way by which the body can, for a short time, keep providing energy for physical activity when oxygen supplies do not meet the needs of the cells. However, if it accumulates throughout the body or in a muscle, it interferes with contraction and fatigue occurs. A trained person can utilize a greater percentage of his or her aerobic power than an untrained person can (see questions 42 and 43) before lactic acid is formed in large quantities.

102. What is intermittent exercise*?*

In intermittent exercise, brief periods of intense activity are interspersed with periods of recovery. If the intense activity is not too long or the recovery period not too short, work can be carried on for a long period of time. By using this concept, it is possible for someone to do high-intensity work within a given period of time. This is one of the principles of interval training.

103. What are contraindicated exercises*?*

Contraindicated exercises are those that, if performed, would put the participant at risk of injury. Recently the number of exercises regarded as contraindicated has seemed to increase even though in many cases the research literature has not shown the exercises to be harmful.

Of course, there will be a significant difference between contraindicated exercises for healthy participants and those for participants with previous or current injuries. Individuals with problems affecting their feet, ankles, knees, hips, lower back, or neck will need to be more careful. For instance, running is contraindicated for someone who has bad knees or lower-back pain but not for most healthy people.

Impact, in particular, has gotten a bad name, especially with the popularization of low-impact aerobics. However, most sports and recreational activities involve impact. Although impact may be undesirable for those who have orthopedic problems (who may participate in safer activities such as swimming and bicycling), it is not innately bad.

104. How does smoking affect the response to exercise?

Smoking increases the oxygen cost of breathing during intense exercise, even in chronic smokers; there is no adaptation to it. The heart-rate response for a given exercise intensity is also greater. In general, smoking prior to exercise decreases the person's maximal capacity.

105. How does the body use adenosine triphosphate (ATP)*, and where is it produced?*

Muscles are powered by the energy released from the breakdown of ATP. The muscles contain very little ATP, and, as it is quickly depleted during muscle work, it must constantly be replaced. This replacement comes from three sources. First, the body cells store small amounts of ATP and creatine phosphate (CP) that are used for energy in short bursts of exercise. They are referred to as the ATP-CP stores.

Second, when muscle glycogen (stored carbohydrate) passes through the glycolysis pathway (changing the stored carbohydrate into a usable form), a high rate of ATP production results, supplying energy for activities lasting between 3 and 5 minutes. As the end product of glycolysis is lactic acid, which inhibits muscle contraction, the length of the activity must be short. This source of ATP is said to be from the lactic acid system.

Finally, most of the ATP that is produced comes from the oxidation of fatty acids and glucose. Although the rate of ATP production is less than that of the ATP-CP or lactic acid systems, the amount of fatty acids and glucose is so plentiful that the supply of ATP can be used for long-duration events. As oxygen is needed to oxidize the glucose and fatty acids, this source of ATP is said to be from the oxygen system.

The YMCA Physical Fitness Test Battery

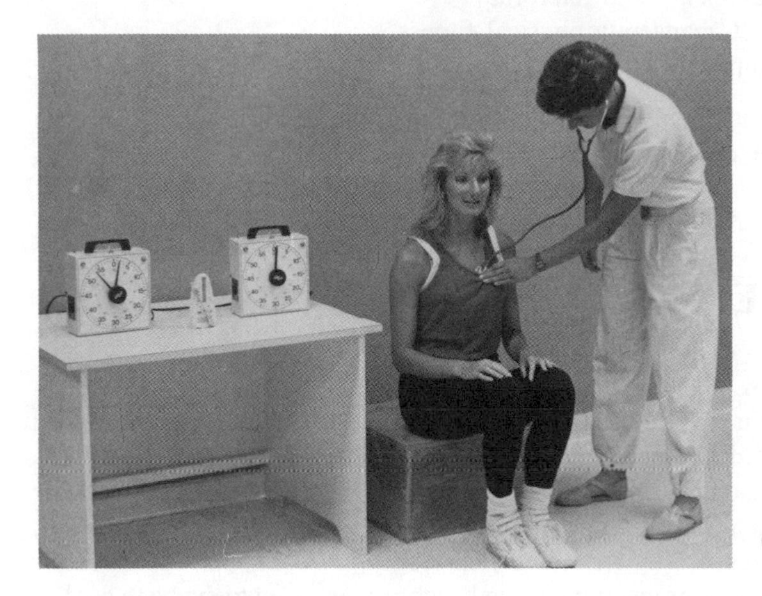

Chapter 4

In a complete physical fitness program, testing and evaluation of participants prior to, during, and after participation are considered important. Reasons for this are to

- assess current fitness levels,
- identify training needs,
- select training regimens,
- evaluate the participant's progress,
- evaluate the success of the program in achieving its objectives, and
- motivate participants.

The evaluation phase of a physical fitness program may be divided into two categories: *medical evaluation* of a participant, which is the responsibility of the individual's physician; and *fitness evaluation*, which is the responsibility of the YMCA fitness director. The medical and fitness evaluations will be covered separately in this chapter.

The sophistication and complexity of a testing program can vary greatly. For many years YMCA fitness programs ranged from no testing at all to testing of practically everything, depending on the individual Y. Most YMCAs are not prepared to utilize tests that require extensive equipment or advanced training for their administration and interpretation. However, every YMCA wants to include tests that offer valid data about the fitness components being measured.

For these reasons the tests selected for the YMCA Physical Fitness Test Battery meet the following criteria:

- Minimal amount of testing time for maximal amount of fitness information
- Within the capability of the physical educator
- Simple to administer and interpret
- Clearly reflect changes in physical fitness
- Minimal equipment expenditure required

Additional tests may be used at the discretion of the local physical education committee and/or medical advisory committee.

MEDICAL EVALUATION VERSUS PHYSICAL FITNESS EVALUATION

The fitness director, the Medical Advisory Committee, and the participant need to understand the difference between medical evaluation and physical fitness evaluation. For years physical educators tested physical fitness before and after training programs to show changes in physical fitness and efficiency. Push-ups, chin-ups, mile runs, agility tests, and step tests were commonly used. However, when the bicycle ergometer and stethoscope were used to evaluate cardiorespiratory fitness, a misinterpretation of the test's purpose often occurred.

Terms such as *stress test*, *exercise test*, *exercise prescription*, and *diagnosis* were used. The result of using these traditionally medical terms was that some individuals misinterpreted the purpose of the test. The present bicycle ergometer test, which replaces many of the running and stepping tests, evaluates cardiorespiratory efficiency by measuring the heart rate while slowly increasing the workloads. The test is given only for evaluation of cardiorespiratory fitness and not for exercise clearance or diagnosis of abnormalities.

The medical evaluation, on the other hand, is for obtaining medical clearance for an individual wishing to engage in a physical fitness program. A trained physician may evaluate the ECG and blood pressure of an individual who is exercising on the bicycle ergometer or treadmill. Along with a medical history, an individual's limitations to exercise, if any, are determined. The tests are used to give medical clearance, diagnose early signs of heart disease, or write an exercise prescription but not to determine the level of cardiovascular fitness. This confusion between physical fitness evaluation and medical clearance needs to be clarified and explained to the medical community, the Medical Advisory Committee, and most of all to the participants.

MEDICAL EVALUATION

The recommendations made for the medical evaluation of an individual are basically the same regardless of the nature of the fitness evaluation format. A medical evaluation is suggested for most national YMCA programs.

The medical examination precedes the physical fitness testing program. The participant's physician is responsible for administering the medical evaluation and giving his or her consent for the participant's further evaluation by the YMCA Physical Fitness Test Battery and for participation in exercise programs. This part of the chapter should be shared with the examining physician.

The American College of Sports Medicine has established guidelines for admitting adults into exercise programs. Emphasis is placed on the age and health status of the proposed participant. Generally, participants are given an exercise stress ECG prior to entering an exercise program for one of the following reasons:

1. To aid in the diagnosis of coronary heart disease in asymptomatic or symptomatic individuals.
2. To assess the safety of exercise prior to starting an exercise program.
3. To assess the cardiopulmonary functional capacity of apparently healthy or diseased individuals.
4. To follow the progress of known coronary or pulmonary disease.
5. To assess the efficacy of various medical and surgical procedures including the effect of medications.*

Categories of Individuals Tested

According to the American College of Sports Medicine, there are three major categories of individuals that may undergo exercise stress ECG testing:

1. Apparently healthy—those who are apparently healthy and have no major coronary risk factors.
2. Individuals at higher risk—those who have symptoms suggestive of possible coronary disease and/or at least one major coronary risk factor (Table 4-1).
3. Individuals with disease—those with known cardiac, pulmonary, or metabolic disease.**

Each of these groups will be discussed briefly.

Apparently Healthy Individuals

Apparently healthy individuals under age 45 can begin a Y's Way to Physical Fitness program because it is based on fitness test assessment results and starts and progresses at an appropriate level. The Y's Way test battery, which is a submaximal test battery, can be given without a physician being present.

Individuals at Higher Risk

Individuals at higher risk are those who display at least one major coronary risk factor (see Table 4-1) and/or symptoms that may be suggestive of cardiopulmonary or metabolic disease.

---

*From *Guidelines for Exercise Testing and Prescription* (3rd ed.) (pp. 1-2) by American College of Sports Medicine, 1986, Philadelphia: Lea & Febiger. Copyright 1986 by Lea & Febiger. Reprinted by permission.

**From *Guidelines for Exercise Testing and Prescription* (3rd ed.) (p. 2) by American College of Sports Medicine, 1986, Philadelphia: Lea & Febiger. Copyright 1986 by Lea & Febiger. Reprinted by permission.

Table 4-1 Major Coronary Risk Factors

1. History of high blood pressure (above 145/95).
2. Elevated total cholesterol/high density lipoprotein cholesterol ratio (above 5).
3. Cigarette smoking.
4. Abnormal resting ECG—including evidence of old myocardial infarction, left ventricular hypertrophy, ischemia, conduction defects, dysrhythmias.
5. Family history of coronary or other atherosclerotic disease prior to age 50.
6. Diabetes mellitus.

Note. From *Guidelines for Exercise Testing and Prescription* (3rd ed.) (p. 2) by American College of Sports Medicine, 1986, Philadelphia: Lea & Febiger. Copyright 1986 by Lea & Febiger. Reprinted by permission.

Individuals With Disease

Individuals at any age who have cardiovascular, pulmonary, or metabolic disease should have medical clearance and exercise stress ECG testing prior to an exercise program. The testing should indicate functional capacity and exercise prescription.

Components of Medical Evaluation

The type and extensiveness of the medical evaluation depends on the physician and the category of the individual participant. The American College of Sports Medicine suggests three major components (medical history, physical examination, and laboratory tests) for the medical evaluation.

Medical History*

This is the most important part of the evaluation. Individuals should be questioned about a history of the following:

A. Heart attack, coronary bypass, or other cardiac surgery
B. Chest discomfort—especially with exertion
C. High blood pressure
D. Extra, skipped, or rapid heart beats/palpitations
E. Heart murmurs, clicks, or unusual cardiac findings
F. Rheumatic fever
G. Ankle swelling
H. Peripheral vascular disease
I. Phlebitis, emboli
J. Unusual shortness of breath
K. Light-headedness or fainting
L. Pulmonary disease including asthma, emphysema and bronchitis

*This section from *Guidelines for Exercise Testing and Prescription* (3rd ed.) (pp. 4-6) by American College of Sports Medicine, 1986, Philadelphia: Lea & Febiger. Copyright 1986 by Lea & Febiger. Reprinted by permission.

M. Abnormal blood lipids

N. Diabetes

O. Stroke

P. Emotional disorders

Q. Medications of all types

R. Recent illness, hospitalization or surgical procedure

S. Drug allergies

T. Orthopedic problems, arthritis

U. Family (grandparents, parents, aunts, uncles, and siblings) history should be explored for the following:
   1. Coronary disease—at what age
   2. Sudden death—at what age
   3. Congenital heart disease

V. Other habits
   1. Caffeine including cola drinks
   2. Alcohol
   3. Tobacco
   4. Other unusual habits or dieting
   5. Exercise history with information on habitual level of activity: type of exercise, frequency, duration, and intensity

Physical Examination*

A limited physical examination is useful to specifically assess:

A. Weight/body composition

B. Orthopedic problems including arthritis

C. Presence of any acute illness

D. Most significant non-cardiac problems which might influence exercise testing and prescription will be identified through the medical history. Areas of possible concern revealed by the history should be evaluated in the physical examination.

E. Cardiovascular evaluation: The following is an adequate cardiac evaluation prior to exercise testing. If a physician is present this cardiovascular evaluation can easily be carried out in minutes. If the evaluation is being conducted when physician presence is not required, then as much of the evaluation as can be carried out competently should be performed.
   1. Pulse rate and regularity
   2. Blood pressure: supine, sitting, and standing
   3. Auscultation of the lungs with specific attention to:
      a. rales, wheezes, and rhonchi
      b. uniformity of breath sounds in all areas

*This section from *Guidelines for Exercise Testing and Prescription* (3rd ed.) (pp. 4-6) by American College of Sports Medicine, 1986, Philadelphia: Lea & Febiger. Copyright 1986 by Lea & Febiger. Reprinted by permission.

4. Palpation for carotid, femoral, and pedal pulses and for cardiac impulse and thrills
5. Auscultation of the heart with specific attention to murmurs, gallops, clicks, and rubs
6. Carotid, abdominal, or femoral bruits
7. Edema
8. Xanthoma and xanthelasma

Laboratory Tests*

Laboratory data are important in the determination of whether an individual fits in the higher risk category. Some laboratory data are helpful prior to testing those with known cardiac, pulmonary, or metabolic disease. The following tests are useful in assessing risk and in assigning individuals to the categories described.

A. Apparently healthy or higher risk individuals
   1. Total cholesterol/high density lipoprotein cholesterol ratio
   2. Triglycerides
   3. Blood glucose
B. Coronary disease
   1. Above tests plus results of all pertinent previous cardiovascular laboratory tests (i.e., angiography, radionuclide studies, previous exercise tests)
   2. Chest X ray
C. Pulmonary disease
   1. Chest X ray
   2. Routine spirometry to include vital capacity and forced expiratory flow volumes
   3. Results of other specialized pulmonary studies

Testing and Exercise Restrictions

Medical clearance and informed-consent forms are required of participants before physical fitness testing and conditioning programs begin. The informed-consent form should include a statement, signed by the participant, that clearly describes both the testing and the exercise program so that the participant is fully aware of what tests will be given and what type of exercise he or she will participate in. Additionally, a statement of the physician's approval for the participant's enrollment in the program should be included. Sample forms are in Appendix D.

The physician, the YMCA Medical Advisory Committee, and the fitness director should also be aware of the relative contraindications to exercise. Individuals having one or more of the contraindications (according to American College of Sports Medicine guidelines) should not be permitted to enter any exercise program that is conducted without medical supervision. Each participant

*This section from *Guidelines for Exercise Testing and Prescription* (3rd ed.) (pp. 4-6) by American College of Sports Medicine, 1986, Philadelphia: Lea & Febiger. Copyright 1986 by Lea & Febiger. Reprinted by permission.

with contraindications should have an individual follow-up in which the benefits of the exercise program are weighed against any resulting harm. Obviously, this demands good clinical judgment. In some instances the participant's condition may not be tangibly altered, but some signs of mental or physical improvement that enhance a sense of well-being may show through. Under such circumstances, the exercise program should be continued even though, from an objective standpoint, the participant's condition appears unchanged.

PHYSICAL FITNESS EVALUATION

After the medical examination has been completed and the medical clearance and informed-consent forms have been received, the participant is ready for the physical fitness evaluation. This evaluation will be done by the YMCA physical fitness specialist. For participants in their first year of training, it is desirable to repeat this test battery after about 10 to 12 weeks and then again after 6 and 12 months. This will show participants their personal response to training. After the first year, most participants need not be tested more than once a year.

Participants should be told the following guidelines before they come for fitness testing:

1. Wear exercise clothing and shoes for the test.
2. Do not eat for 2 hours before testing (this includes drinking coffee or tea).
3. Do not consume alcohol for 24 hours before testing.
4. Do not smoke for 2 hours before testing.
5. Do not exercise on the day of testing.

The four areas of physical fitness selected for evaluation are body composition, cardiorespiratory endurance, flexibility, and muscular strength and endurance. The tests are administered in the following order:

1. Standing height (if taken)
2. Weight
3. Resting heart rate
4. Resting blood pressure
5. Body composition
6. Cardiovascular evaluation
7. Flexibility measurement
8. Muscular strength and endurance

The test results should be recorded on the score sheet for men or the score sheet for women at the end of this chapter. Be sure to complete the demographic information at the top of the score sheet. Results can then be transferred to the Body Composition Profile and Physical Fitness Evaluation Profile forms that also appear at the end of this chapter. The Physical Fitness Evaluation Profile form rates all results on a scale from *excellent* to *very poor*.

The remainder of this chapter will cover the testing procedures, beginning with some standard measurements.

Standard Measurements

Measurements of height, weight, and resting heart rate and blood pressure provide a baseline for measuring improvement and evaluating changes. Follow these procedures to record them.

STANDING HEIGHT: The participant should stand barefoot with the heels together, then stretch upward to the fullest extent. Heels, buttocks, and upper back should touch a vertical upright such as a wall. The chin should not be lifted. Measurement is recorded in inches to the nearest quarter inch. (Because this is not a physical fitness measurement, it may be eliminated. It is a good description of the participant and is easy to administer.)

WEIGHT: Weight should be recorded with the individual wearing gym shorts, T-shirt, and no shoes. Make note of any deviation from this dress. Record weight in both pounds and kilograms. Record to the nearest quarter pound.

RESTING HEART RATE: The resting heart rate should be counted through the use of a stethoscope for 1 minute. The individual should be sitting (as for a blood pressure test) and should have had an adequate rest period prior to this test. Adequate rest is indicated when the heart rate has stabilized at a low rate and has not changed.

RESTING BLOOD PRESSURE: The individual sits upright in a straight-backed chair. Both feet are flat on the floor, and the left arm is resting on a table with the elbow flexed. The position is relaxed and comfortable, and the individual is allowed to relax for a few minutes in this position. Conversation is discouraged. The blood pressure is measured with a device called a sphygmomanometer and with a stethoscope. A wide, adjustable cuff is placed around the subject's upper left arm approximately at heart level. Air is pumped into this cuff, which then expands and presses against the arm to close off the brachial artery, which runs along the inside of the arm. The pressure in the cuff is shown by the sphygmomanometer in millimeters of mercury and initially is pumped up to 200 mm Hg, which is normally higher than the individual's blood pressure. The stethoscope is placed in the antecubital space below the cuff. Once the brachial artery has been closed off, air is slowly released from the cuff, and the tester listens for the moment at which the resumption of blood flow can be heard. This resumed flow is characterized by a distinctive sound and is called the systolic pressure. The pressure in the cuff is further reduced until blood runs freely through the artery. This point is characterized by the complete disappearance of sound and is called diastolic pressure. There are three intermediary phases of subtle changes that are not of concern here. The first phase—systolic pressure—and the fifth—diastolic pressure—should be recorded in millimeters of mercury (mm Hg) as indicated on the sphygmomanometer scale.

Body Composition

Body composition refers to the lean body weight plus the fat weight, which together make up total body weight. The measurement of body composition is important, as obesity is a known health hazard. Obesity is related to a higher incidence of numerous diseases, including coronary heart disease, diabetes, cirrhosis of the liver, hernia, and intestinal obstruction. Obesity is also of considerable concern from an aesthetic standpoint and may be one of the primary reasons an individual decides to join a YMCA exercise program. Therefore, it is important to be able to identify an individual's initial body composition before training and also to quantify any change that may occur with training and/or diet. A desirable weight should be determined for the individual, but reducing weight alone should not be the only goal.

Gross weight is not a good measurement of body composition. Height and weight tables are limited, as what makes up the weight is not taken into consideration. One person 6 ft tall and weighing 200 lb may be "overweight," whereas another person with the same measurement may be "normal." If the added pounds are fat, this is considered undesirable; however, if the weight is muscle mass, as in a bodybuilder, the extra pounds are normal and desirable.

Methods of Determining Desirable Weight

There are a number of ways to determine what a fit individual should weigh. Some assign a weight on the basis of norms and others on the basis of desirable percentage of fat to total body weight. Each method has both benefits and drawbacks. The most common methods follow.

Height and Weight Tables

These tables have the major limitation of not distinguishing among bone, muscle, and fat. A case demonstrating this limitation occurred at a large metropolitan police department that had height and weight limitations for its officers (which now are considered discriminatory). The maximum allowable weight for a 6-ft officer was 210 lb; above this weight an officer was considered overweight and subject to suspension. Two officers were suspended for being 6 ft tall and over 210 lb; both were bodybuilders and had only 19% fat. Considerable explanation was needed to reinstate the officers. This case clearly illustrates the limitations of height and weight tables.

Tables have been improved by allowing for variations in small, average, and large frames and removing the factors that permitted an increase in weight with age. Because bone and muscle growth is complete when one reaches adulthood, increases in weight with age have to be undesirable fat. The same standards are now used for everyone over 25 years of age.

The benefits of the tables are speed and familiarity. These tables were constructed from data on thousands of people and thus represent good averages. They can still be used by someone of average build.

Skinfold Measurements

When individuals gain fat, much of this added adipose tissue occurs in subcutaneous areas in certain parts of the body. This subcutaneous fat can be pinched up by the thumb and forefingers; as individuals get fatter, these skinfolds get larger.

Skinfold calipers have been designed to measure the thickness of this skin and subcutaneous fat. The medical calipers are designed with a constant tension spring so that, regardless of how wide the caliper jaws spread, the tension between the jaws is constant (see Figs. 4-1 and 4-2). However, there is a difference in jaw pressure between different makes of calipers and care should be taken to only test with one make when doing fitness evaluations.

Skinfold measurements are excellent estimates of total body fat. Norm tables are included in this chapter to determine average, below average, or above

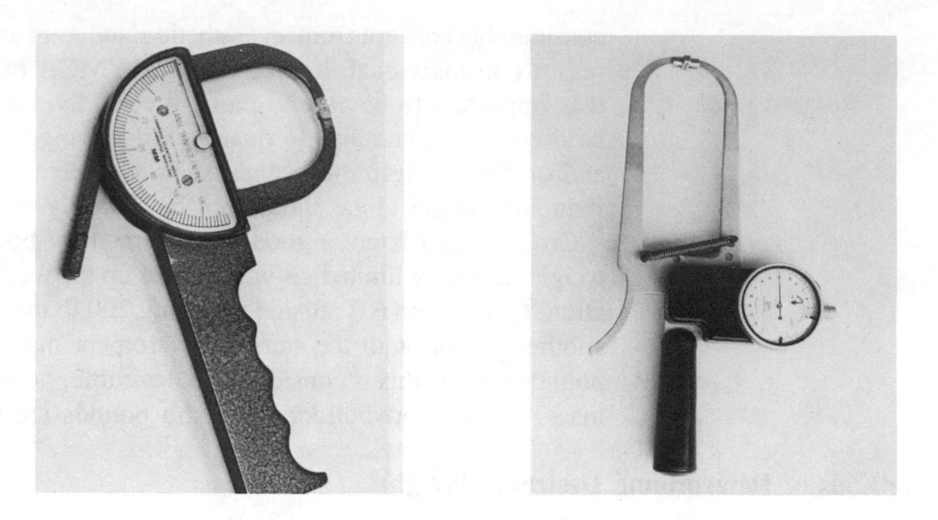

Figure 4-1. Lange skinfold caliper. **Figure 4-2.** Harpenden skinfold caliper.

average ratings. These measurements also correlate very well with more sophisticated determinations of body fat. Skinfold measurements require only skinfold calipers and practice to be reliable and valid.

Considerable practice of skinfold measurement is needed for accuracy, and those who use this method should practice on a group of individuals over and over again, recording the measurements until results become consistent. Consistency can be checked by having the same individual measured by two different testers; the difference should not exceed 2 millimeters (mm). If the difference exceeds 2 mm, more practice is needed to standardize the procedure. A coefficient of correlation can be computed on each skinfold location by a simple test/retest procedure of about 20 participants. This procedure is explained in standard test and measurement textbooks and is also programmed on some inexpensive hand-held calculators.

Skinfold test locations are those sites where fat usually accumulates. Details on sites and measurement techniques are given later in this section.

The benefits of skinfold measurements are obvious. Little equipment is needed, they can be done quickly, and the interpretation is simple. An individual who has an abdominal skinfold of 28 mm at the start of a program and reduces this to 18 mm in 20 weeks has a reduction of 10 mm in the measurement, or 5 mm of fat at this site (a skinfold is two thicknesses of skin). It is not uncommon to add the measurements at the various sites and call this amount the *total fat*. Caution should be used in comparing total fat measurements to norm tables; be sure that the norm tables use the same sites and the same number of sites.

The major disadvantage of skinfold testing is that too many individuals use the calipers with insufficient practice. Caliper measurements are not reliable when first taken but do become very reliable with adequate practice.

Circumference Measurements*

Because skinfold measurements require a high level of expertise resulting from practice and tested reliability, it is difficult to find trained technicians capable of capturing consistent measurements. A simple alternative method for predicting percent body fat has been developed using easily measured body circumfer-

*From ''A Comparative Review of Four Methods for Calculating Percent Body Fat'' by J. Donahue, L. Golding, and L. Cummings, 1988, *Perspective*, **14**, p. 34. Copyright 1988 by Joseph Donahue, Lawrence Golding, and Leslie Cummings. Reprinted by permission.

ences together with height, weight, and age data. Large numbers of subjects can be measured in a short time, and the only equipment needed is a measuring tape and a weight scale.

McArdle, Katch, and Katch (1981) have developed equations for calculating percent fat by using three circumferences for four population groups: men between 17 and 26 years old, women between 17 and 26, men between 27 and 50, and women between 27 and 50. From the analysis of the data obtained from circumference measurements and underwater weighing, equations have been developed from which percent body fat can be estimated within 2.5% to 4% of the values obtained by the most accurate method of measurement—underwater weighing (discussed later). This is quite acceptable for most screening purposes.

Although the accuracy of estimating percent body fat by skinfold measurements and circumference measurements is similar, many investigators still prefer skinfolds. Skinfolds measure fat directly; whereas circumferences make no distinction between fat and muscle. Circumference measurements are most accurate when subjects are within an average body-fat range. In an extreme case, using circumference to measure someone with a large amount of muscle mass such as a bodybuilder would probably yield an estimated percentage of fat similar to that of an obese person. However, although the obese person might have the same physical size, he or she would have a much greater percentage of body fat than would the bodybuilder.

The anatomical sites selected for measurement vary and may include the circumferences of the abdomen, right thigh, right forearm, right calf, right upper arm, and buttocks. The U.S. Navy is presently using two circumferences to estimate percent fat: the umbilicus and the neck.

Bioelectrical Impedance Analysis (BIA)*

Due in part to a demand for faster and easier methods of evaluation, bioelectrical impedance analysis (BIA) has become a widely used method of estimating percent body fat. The method was originally used in health clubs and spas but is now being used more frequently in medical clinics.

The use of BIA is based on the principle that the conductivity of an electrical impulse is greater through fat-free tissue than it is through fatty tissue. Through electrodes on the hand and foot, the instrument can measure a small electrical current passing between the electrodes and therefore the body's impedance (resistance) to the electrical current in ohms. This ohmmeter is connected to a computer that calculates body density using a series of algebraic equations (a constant multiplied by the weight and the resistance divided by the square of the height). The density is converted to percent body fat using the same equations used with the underwater weighing method.

Keying on the figure obtained for percent body fat, the BIA computer can provide printouts for a variety of information specific to each individual, including the percent and absolute amount of body fat, total body water, and lean body weight. Optional printouts can include nutrition tables, diet and exercise programs, energy-expenditure charts, and suggested weight-loss/weight-gain charts.

The attractiveness and marketability of BIA are its speed (about 3 minutes per subject), ease of operation, and self-explanatory computer printouts. Participant compliance with suggestions to improve health is boosted by the ''print-out

*From ''A Comparative Review of Four Methods for Calculating Percent Body Fat'' by J. Donahue, L. Golding, and L. Cummings, 1988, *Perspective,* **14**, p. 34. Copyright 1988 by Joseph Donahue, Lawrence Golding, and Leslie Cummings. Reprinted by permission.

mystique,'' the belief that computers are infallible. The provider's image may also benefit by association with this very visible high-tech equipment.

However, the output of a computer is no more accurate than its input. In the case of BIA, as the assumptions and formulas used in the computer program are not valid, many of the parameters printed out may have a poor relationship to what was measured. The validity and reliability of BIA is being studied. The first research largely documents the shortcomings of the BIA method. McArdle et al. (1981) found an overestimation of body fat in absolute terms of 6.79% in young males. Scientific papers presented at the 1985 annual meeting of the American College of Sports Medicine showed both overestimations and underestimations of percent body fat for various populations. In most of these studies the body-fat estimations were calculated using the software supplied by the manufacturer of the instruments. Currently a study is being conducted nationally to develop better formulas specific to populations for estimations of percent body fat using BIA.

Other disadvantages of BIA at this time are the initial equipment costs and the time and care required to fit each person with electrodes.

Underwater Weighing*

Underwater, or hydrostatic, weighing is used to determine body density. The method is based on the physics principle that mass divided by volume equals density. Weight is substituted for mass, and volume is either measured directly (volumetric method) or calculated from Archimedes' Principle, which states that the weight a body loses underwater equals the weight of the water it displaces. From this, one can calculate the volume of the water displaced, which equals the volume of the subject. For example, if a 70-kg man weighs 5 kg underwater, then his body has displaced 65 kg, or 65 L, of water. His density is 1.08 g/mL (70 ÷ 65).

Two corrections need to be applied when using density. First, the density of water changes with temperature, thus affecting the calculation of the volume of water displaced. Second, any air in the body needs to be subtracted from underwater weight. There are two sources of air in the body: air in the gastrointestinal tract and residual air in the lungs. Gastrointestinal air is estimated to be approximately 100 mL; this small amount is dropped from most calculations. However, the lung residual volume is significant and must be measured to correct the underwater weight.

Usually underwater weighing is done after the subject has exhaled maximally so that only residual volume needs to be measured. However, if both residual volume and vital capacity are measured, then the subject can be weighed following a maximal inspiration, and the underwater weight can be corrected for total lung volume.

Residual volume and vital capacity can be measured either at the time of weighing (while the person is submerged) or prior to the weighing. Several studies have investigated the validity of determining pulmonary volumes in and out of the water, especially as affected by body position and water pressure on the thorax. Some studies suggest that errors exist when the lung volume measured out of the water is used for correction, as there may be a significant decrease in residual volume and total lung capacity when subjects are submerged. Other

---

*From ''A Comparative Review of Four Methods for Calculating Percent Body Fat'' by J. Donahue, L. Golding, and L. Cummings, 1988, *Perspective*, **14**, p. 34. Copyright 1988 by Joseph Donahue, Lawrence Golding, and Leslie Cummings. Reprinted by permission.

studies find differences in calculated body density when using residual volume and not total lung volume.

Nonswimmers are often apprehensive when submerged in water, and this feeling can be increased when they are asked to exhale maximally. Inexperienced, nervous people may not maximally exhale underwater; thus, if residual volume were measured prior to entering the tank, this would result in inaccurate densities.

Error may occur when density obtained from underwater weighing is used to derive percent body fat. The commonly used calculations are based on assumptions that the density of lean body weight is constant among all people. Several equations are available to estimate percent body fat once the density is determined (see Siri, 1956; Brozek, Grande, Anderson, & Keys, 1963). However, Wilmore (1983) warns that the variability of lean-body-weight density can make these equations inappropriate, especially for younger (8 to 12 years old) and older (72 to 74 years old) males.

The degree of precision of the weighing apparatus used can greatly affect the accuracy of underwater weighing. Many systems use a spring-loaded scale for measuring weight underwater. Even with damping, this type of scale does not stabilize during weighing, so the technician must estimate the weight from a moving scale. Load cells or strain gauges with electronic outputs to a printer or plotter record the weight more accurately.

Although percent fat is only an estimate from the density obtained from underwater weighing, it is still the best available estimate. Underwater weighing's potential error of 2.5% is considered minimal. Although it has limitations, underwater weighing is the benchmark for validating other methods. It is the "gold standard" for estimating percent body fat.

Prediction Equations

Prediction equations are statistical procedures for estimating body composition from simple anthropometrical measurements. The results are validated by comparison to hydrostatic weighing.

There are several prediction equations in the research literature, and many have proven to be highly reliable and valid. Because these predictions are taken from measurements on certain populations, they are usually accurate only when applied to a similar population. Therefore, equations have been published for young boys, young recruits in the army, adult males, high school girls, and adult women. Calculation usually involves using one or more of a number of equations, depending on the population being measured.

Jackson and Pollock (1978) published an equation based on measurements from 403 adult men between the ages of 18 and 61. They found that a limitation on many of the previously published equations was that the slopes of the various regression lines for the various groups were not parallel. This difference resulted in biased body-density estimates. Their studies have shown that the relationship between skinfold measurements and body density is not linear but curvilinear.

The Jackson-Pollock study divided 403 subjects into a validation group of 308 and a cross-validation group of 95. Body density was determined by hydrostatic weighing. Regression analysis was used to derive the generalized equation. Polynomial models were used to test whether the relationship between body density and the sum of skinfolds was curvilinear. This showed that the relationship between skinfold fat and body density was quadratic. Age was used as an independent variable and eliminated the need for several age-adjusted equations. A study of women developed equations that exhibited similar statistical characteristics. A further discussion of this equation is found in the section on estimating percent body fat.

Percent Body Fat and Target Weight

All but one of the preceding procedures result in the estimation of percent body fat. If the percent body fat is known, then a predicted desirable weight can be computed, as it is defined as the lean body weight plus a desirable percentage of fat. Predicted weight may be better termed *target weight*, as the desired weight for different groups may change. Marathon runners may wish to be 10% to 12% fat (as many marathon runners are), whereas weightlifters or football players may prefer to be 19% to 20% fat.

It has been suggested that from a health standpoint men should be 16% fat. This may be a little low for the average male. Males should, however, be under 20% fat and, from an aesthetic and training standpoint, be 16% fat or less. Females should be 23% fat or less. While standards may differ from one laboratory to another, a male over 25% fat and a female over 35% fat would certainly be considered to have marginal obesity. The new norms collected on 20,000 Y members show that men average between 15% and 25%, and women average between 25% and 32%.

Those who are obese should be warned of the potential health hazards of obesity and the desirability of bringing one's weight within a more normal range. The fitness director could recommend, in consultation with a physician, a program of diet and exercise that would produce a gradual weight loss. Crash diets are unwise from a health standpoint and are rarely successful in keeping weight off. A realistic goal is a caloric deficit, obtained through a diet and exercise regimen, of no more than 500 Kcal per day, continuing until the desired weight is achieved. It should be remembered in recommending exercise for an overweight individual that practically all work is more difficult due to the excess weight, and consideration must be given to the type and intensity of exercise that can be tolerated by this person.

The computation of target weight is accomplished after the determination of percent fat. The method described later in this chapter results in a percent fat for a certain age. After this is determined, a target weight is computed as follows:

EXAMPLE 1: Subject A: male, 40 years old, weighs 210 lb. He is 23% fat as determined by the Jackson-Pollock equation.

a. If 23% of his weight is fat, his fat weight in pounds is determined by calculating 23% of his total weight (23% of 210 lb = 48.3 lb of fat).

b. Subtracting his fat weight from his total weight will give his lean body weight (LBW): 210 − 48.3 = 161.7. Without fat his body weight is 161.7 lb.

c. Instead of 23% fat, he should be 16% fat. This is obtained by taking his LBW (161.7) and adding 16% fat: LBW/.84 = weight at 16% fat, or 161.7/.84 = 192.5 lb. (.84 is 100% − 16%.)

Table 4-2 allows this figure to be determined without computation. Actual weight (210) is found along the top of the table, percent fat (23%) is found along the left-hand side, and where these two intersect is the target weight (193 lb) at 16%. (This would be 192.5 lb if computed as shown above.)

Table 4-2 Target Weight—Men (16% Fat)

	Body weight (lb)																								
% fat	120	125	130	135	140	145	150	155	160	165	170	175	180	185	190	195	200	205	210	215	220	225	230	235	240
17	119	123	129	133	138	143	148	153	158	163	168	173	179	183	188	193	198	203	208	212	217	222	227	232	237
18	117	122	127	132	137	142	146	151	156	161	166	171	176	181	186	190	195	200	205	210	215	220	225	229	234
19	116	121	125	130	135	140	145	149	154	159	164	169	174	178	183	188	193	198	203	207	212	217	222	225	231
20	114	119	124	129	133	138	143	148	152	157	162	167	171	176	181	186	190	195	200	205	210	214	219	224	229
21	113	118	122	127	132	136	141	146	150	155	160	165	169	174	179	183	188	193	198	202	207	212	216	221	226
22	111	116	121	125	130	135	139	144	149	153	158	162	167	172	176	181	186	190	195	200	204	209	214	218	223
23	110	115	119	123	128	133	138	142	147	151	156	160	165	170	174	179	183	188	193	197	202	206	211	215	220
24	109	113	118	122	127	131	136	140	145	149	154	158	163	167	172	176	181	186	190	195	199	204	208	213	217
25	107	112	116	121	125	129	134	138	143	147	152	156	161	165	170	174	179	183	188	192	196	201	205	210	214
26	106	110	115	119	123	128	132	137	141	145	150	154	159	163	167	172	176	181	185	189	194	198	203	207	211
27	104	109	113	117	122	126	130	135	139	143	148	152	156	161	165	169	174	178	183	187	191	196	200	204	209
28	103	107	111	116	120	124	129	133	137	141	146	150	154	159	163	167	171	176	180	184	189	193	197	201	208
29	101	106	110	114	118	123	127	131	135	139	144	148	152	156	161	165	169	173	178	182	186	190	194	199	203
30	100	104	108	113	117	121	125	129	133	137	142	146	150	154	158	162	167	171	175	179	183	188	192	196	200
31	99	103	107	111	115	119	123	127	131	136	140	144	149	152	156	160	164	168	173	177	181	185	189	193	197
32	97	101	105	109	113	117	121	125	130	134	138	142	146	150	154	158	162	166	170	174	178	182	186	190	194
33	96	100	104	108	112	116	120	124	128	132	136	140	144	148	152	156	160	164	168	171	175	179	183	187	191
34	94	98	102	106	110	114	118	122	126	130	134	137	141	145	149	153	157	161	165	169	173	177	181	185	189
35	93	97	101	104	108	112	116	120	124	128	132	135	139	143	147	151	155	159	163	166	170	174	178	182	186
36	91	95	99	103	107	110	114	118	122	126	130	133	137	141	145	149	152	156	160	164	168	171	175	179	183
37	90	94	98	101	105	109	113	116	120	124	128	131	135	139	143	146	150	154	158	161	165	169	173	176	180
38	89	92	96	100	103	107	111	114	118	122	125	129	133	137	140	144	148	151	155	159	162	166	170	174	177
39	87	91	94	98	102	105	109	112	116	120	123	127	131	134	138	142	145	149	153	156	160	163	167	171	174
40	86	89	93	96	100	104	107	111	114	118	121	125	129	132	136	139	143	146	150	154	157	161	164	168	173

Note. To use, find the subject's present weight at the top of the table, then descend vertically to the horizontal row corresponding to the estimated percent fat. For example, the target weight for a man who weighed 210 lb and was 23% fat would be 193 lb (see text for computation).

EXAMPLE 2: Subject B: female, 35 years old, weight 145 lb. She is 28% fat as determined by the Jackson-Pollock equation.

a. If 28% of her weight is fat, her fat weight in pounds is determined by calculating 28% of her total weight (28% of 145 lb = 40.6 lb of fat).

b. Subtracting this fat weight from total weight will give her LBW: 145 − 40.6 = 104.4 lb. Without fat her body weight is 104.4 lb.

c. Instead of 28% fat she should be 23% fat. This is obtained by taking her LBW (104.4) and adding 23% fat: LBW/.77 = weight at 23% fat, or 104.4/.77 = 135.6 lb. Table 4-3 allows this to be done without computation.

Occasionally a person will be measured whose percent fat is lower than the norm. This has sometimes caused concern in interpretation. For example, if a male subject is 12% fat as determined by the Jackson-Pollock equation and weighs 167 lb, this should not be interpreted as a need to gain 4%. The target weight is based on the general population. This individual should be told that he is in the range of very fit marathon runners and that it is often desirable to be under the norm; most athletes are. This is the reason that Tables 4-2 and 4-3 do not go under 17% and 24%, respectively.

Estimation of Body Fat by Skinfolds

The YMCA's method of estimating body fat involves the measurement of skinfolds in various body locations. A number of equations have been developed for specific populations (e.g., young or old, male or female, active or sedentary individuals) and may not be used interchangeably. The equation selected for this book is based on the research of Jackson and Pollock (1978) and has been shown to be a valid and reliable. Because the YMCA had specific problems with certain skinfold sites, Jackson adapted the research and developed equations specifically for the YMCA.

The actual equation and statistics are not necessary for the user but are presented on the facing page for those interested. Tables based on the sums of skinfold measurements and on age are included in this chapter to allow direct readings in percent fat.

Both men and women use the sum of four sites: abdomen, ilium, tricep, and thigh. As experience has shown that accurate measurement of the thigh is sometimes difficult, Jackson constructed additional tables that eliminate the thigh measurement. The equations based on the sum of three sites (abdomen, ilium, and tricep) should be used only if the thigh skinfold cannot be measured accurately.

The fitness director should attempt to measure the four skinfold sites and use Table 4-4 for men and Table 4-5 for women. If the thigh measurement cannot be taken or appears inaccurate, then the sum of three sites should be used with Tables 4-6 and 4-7. Two examples of finding the target weight with four skinfold site measurements follow.

FOUR SITES

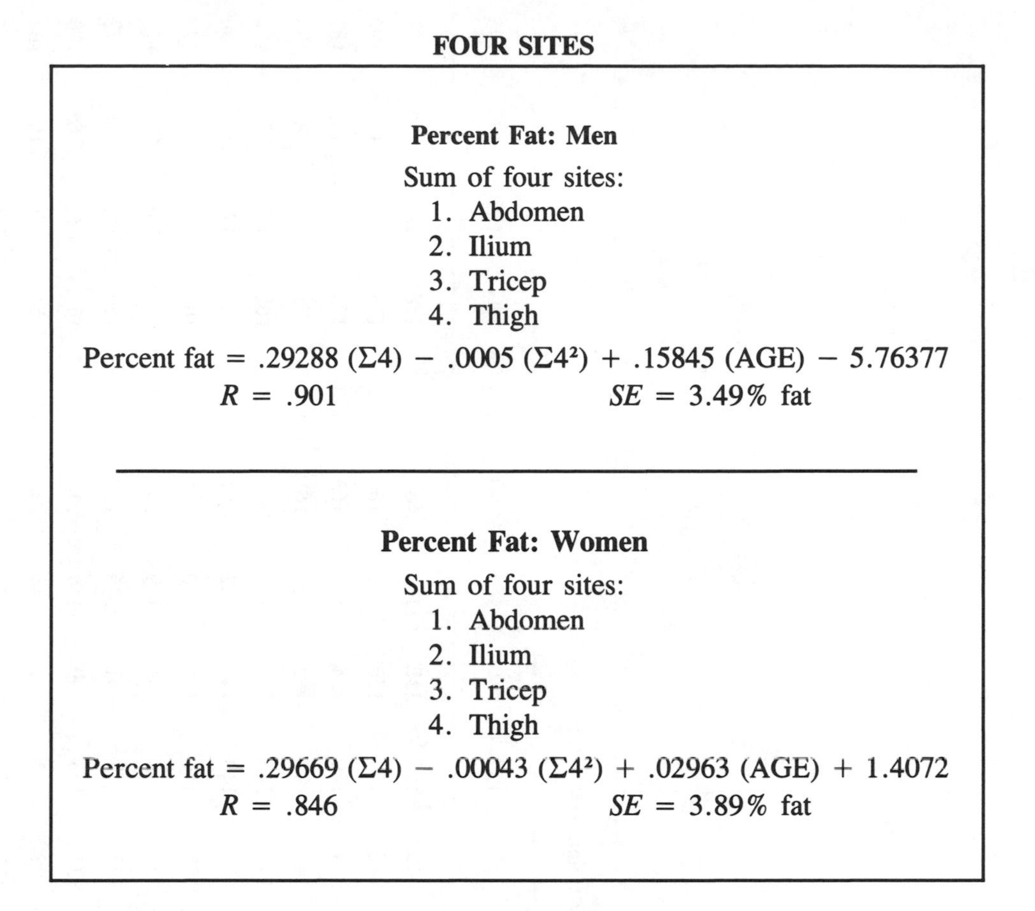

Percent Fat: Men

Sum of four sites:

1. Abdomen
2. Ilium
3. Tricep
4. Thigh

$$\text{Percent fat} = .29288\,(\Sigma 4) - .0005\,(\Sigma 4^2) + .15845\,(\text{AGE}) - 5.76377$$

$R = .901$ $SE = 3.49\%$ fat

Percent Fat: Women

Sum of four sites:

1. Abdomen
2. Ilium
3. Tricep
4. Thigh

$$\text{Percent fat} = .29669\,(\Sigma 4) - .00043\,(\Sigma 4^2) + .02963\,(\text{AGE}) + 1.4072$$

$R = .846$ $SE = 3.89\%$ fat

THREE SITES

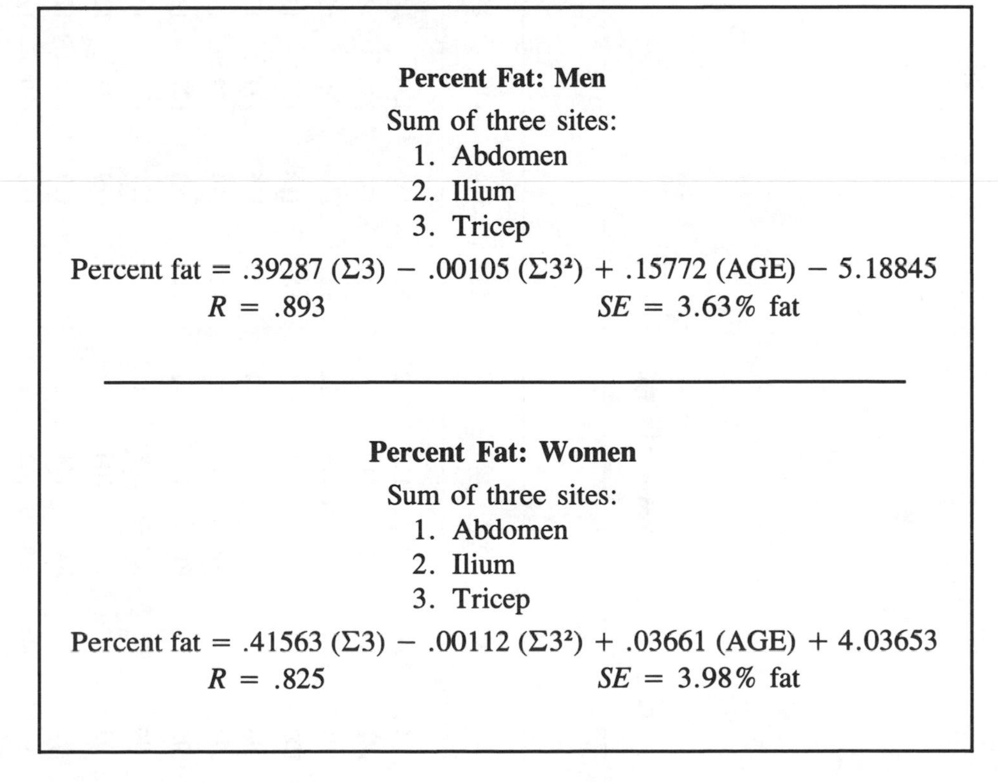

Percent Fat: Men

Sum of three sites:

1. Abdomen
2. Ilium
3. Tricep

$$\text{Percent fat} = .39287\,(\Sigma 3) - .00105\,(\Sigma 3^2) + .15772\,(\text{AGE}) - 5.18845$$

$R = .893$ $SE = 3.63\%$ fat

Percent Fat: Women

Sum of three sites:

1. Abdomen
2. Ilium
3. Tricep

$$\text{Percent fat} = .41563\,(\Sigma 3) - .00112\,(\Sigma 3^2) + .03661\,(\text{AGE}) + 4.03653$$

$R = .825$ $SE = 3.98\%$ fat

Table 4-3 Target Weight—Women (23% Fat)

%	Body weight (lb)																		
fat	105	110	115	120	125	130	135	140	145	150	155	160	165	170	175	180	185	190	195
24	104	109	114	118	123	128	133	138	143	148	153	158	163	168	173	178	183	188	192
25	102	107	112	117	122	127	131	136	141	146	151	156	161	166	170	175	180	185	190
26	101	106	111	115	120	125	130	135	139	144	149	154	159	163	168	173	178	183	187
27	100	104	109	114	119	123	128	133	137	142	147	152	156	161	166	171	175	180	185
28	98	103	108	112	117	122	126	131	136	140	145	150	154	159	164	168	173	178	182
29	97	101	106	111	115	120	124	129	134	138	143	148	152	157	161	166	171	175	180
30	95	100	105	109	114	118	123	127	132	136	141	145	150	155	159	164	168	173	177
31	94	99	103	108	112	116	121	125	130	134	139	144	149	152	157	161	166	170	175
32	93	97	102	106	110	115	119	124	129	132	137	141	146	150	155	159	163	168	172
33	91	96	100	104	109	113	117	122	126	131	135	139	144	148	152	157	161	165	170
34	90	94	99	103	107	111	116	120	124	129	133	137	141	146	150	154	159	163	167
35	89	93	97	101	106	110	114	118	122	127	131	135	139	144	148	152	156	160	165
36	87	91	96	100	104	108	112	116	121	125	129	133	137	141	145	150	154	158	162
37	86	90	94	98	102	106	110	115	119	123	127	131	135	139	143	147	151	155	160
38	85	89	93	97	101	105	109	113	117	121	125	129	133	137	141	145	149	153	157
39	83	87	91	95	99	103	107	111	115	119	123	127	131	135	139	143	147	151	154
40	82	86	90	94	97	101	105	109	113	117	121	125	129	132	136	140	144	148	152

Note. To use, find the subject's present weight at the top of the table, then descend vertically to the horizontal row corresponding to the estimated percent fat. For example, the target weight for a woman who weighed 145 lb and was 28% fat would be 136 lb (see text for computation.)

Table 4-4 Percent Fat Estimates for Four Sites—Men

	Age to last year								
Sum of 4 skinfolds	18-22	23-27	28-32	33-37	38-42	43-47	48-52	53-57	≥ 58
13-17	1.7	2.5	3.3	4.1	4.9	5.6	6.4	7.2	8.0
18-22	3.1	3.9	4.6	5.4	6.2	7.0	7.8	8.6	9.4
23-27	4.4	5.2	6.0	6.8	7.6	8.4	9.2	10.0	10.7
28-32	5.7	6.5	7.3	8.1	8.9	9.7	10.5	11.3	12.1
33-37	7.0	7.8	8.6	9.4	10.2	11.0	11.8	12.6	13.4
38-42	8.3	9.1	9.9	10.7	11.5	12.3	13.1	13.9	14.6
43-47	9.6	10.3	11.1	11.9	12.7	13.5	14.3	15.1	15.9
48-52	10.8	11.6	12.4	13.2	13.9	14.7	15.5	16.3	17.1
53-57	12.0	12.8	13.6	14.4	15.1	15.9	16.7	17.5	18.3
58-62	13.1	13.9	14.7	15.5	16.3	17.1	17.9	18.7	19.5
63-67	14.3	15.1	15.9	16.7	17.5	18.2	19.0	19.8	20.6
68-72	15.4	16.2	17.0	17.8	18.6	19.4	20.2	21.0	21.8
73-77	16.5	17.3	18.1	18.9	19.7	20.5	21.3	22.1	22.8
78-82	17.6	18.4	19.2	20.0	20.7	21.5	22.3	23.1	23.9
83-87	18.6	19.4	20.2	21.0	21.8	22.6	23.4	24.2	25.0
88-92	19.6	20.4	21.2	22.0	22.8	23.6	24.4	25.2	26.0
93-97	20.6	21.4	22.2	23.0	23.8	24.6	25.4	26.2	27.0
98-102	21.6	22.4	23.2	24.0	24.8	25.6	26.4	27.1	27.9
103-107	22.5	23.3	24.1	24.9	25.7	26.5	27.3	28.1	28.9
108-112	23.5	24.2	25.0	25.8	26.6	27.4	28.2	29.0	29.8
113-117	24.3	25.1	25.9	26.7	27.5	28.3	29.1	29.9	30.7
118-122	25.2	26.0	26.8	27.6	28.4	29.2	30.0	30.8	31.6
123-127	26.0	26.8	27.6	28.4	29.2	30.0	30.8	31.6	32.4
128-132	26.9	27.7	28.4	29.2	30.0	30.8	31.6	32.4	33.2
133-137	27.7	28.4	29.2	30.0	30.8	31.6	32.4	33.2	34.0
138-142	28.4	29.2	30.0	30.8	31.6	32.4	33.2	34.0	34.8
143-147	29.2	29.9	30.7	31.5	32.3	33.1	33.9	34.7	35.5
148-152	29.9	30.7	31.5	32.2	33.0	33.8	34.6	35.4	36.2
153-157	30.6	31.3	32.1	32.9	33.7	34.5	35.3	36.1	36.9
158-162	31.2	32.0	32.8	33.6	34.4	35.2	36.0	36.8	37.6
163-167	31.8	32.6	33.4	34.2	35.0	35.8	36.6	37.4	38.2
168-172	32.5	33.3	34.0	34.8	35.6	36.4	37.2	38.0	38.8
173-177	33.0	33.8	34.6	35.4	36.2	37.0	37.8	38.6	39.4
178-182	33.6	34.4	35.2	36.0	36.8	37.6	38.4	39.2	39.9
183-187	34.1	34.9	35.7	36.5	37.3	38.1	38.9	39.7	40.5

Table 4-5 Percent Fat Estimates for Four Sites—Women

Sum of 4 skinfolds	Age to last year								
	18-22	23-27	28-32	33-37	38-42	43-47	48-52	53-57	⩾ 58
23-27	8.6	9.3	9.4	9.6	9.7	9.9	10.0	10.2	10.3
28-32	10.0	10.7	10.8	11.0	11.0	11.3	11.4	11.6	11.7
33-37	11.3	12.0	12.2	12.3	12.4	12.6	12.7	12.9	13.0
38-42	12.6	13.3	13.5	13.6	13.7	13.9	14.1	14.2	14.4
43-47	13.9	14.6	14.8	14.9	15.0	15.2	15.4	15.5	15.7
48-52	15.2	15.9	16.1	16.2	16.3	16.5	16.7	16.8	17.0
53-57	16.5	17.2	17.3	17.5	17.5	17.8	17.9	18.1	18.2
58-62	17.7	18.4	18.6	18.7	18.8	19.0	19.1	19.3	19.4
63-67	18.9	19.6	19.8	19.9	20.0	20.2	20.4	20.5	20.7
68-72	20.1	20.8	21.0	21.1	21.2	21.4	21.6	21.7	21.9
73-77	21.3	22.0	22.1	22.3	22.3	22.6	22.7	22.9	23.0
78-82	22.5	23.1	23.3	23.4	23.5	23.7	23.9	24.0	24.2
83-87	23.6	24.3	24.4	24.6	24.6	24.9	25.0	25.2	25.3
88-92	24.7	25.4	25.5	25.7	25.7	26.0	26.1	26.3	26.4
93-97	25.8	26.5	26.6	26.8	26.8	27.1	27.2	27.4	27.5
98-102	26.8	27.5	27.7	27.8	27.9	28.1	28.3	28.4	28.6
103-107	27.9	28.6	28.7	28.9	28.9	29.2	29.3	29.5	29.6
108-112	28.9	29.6	29.7	29.9	30.0	30.2	30.3	30.5	30.6
113-117	29.9	30.6	30.7	30.9	31.0	31.2	31.3	31.5	31.6
118-122	30.9	31.6	31.7	31.9	31.9	32.2	32.3	32.5	32.6
123-127	31.9	32.5	32.7	32.8	32.9	33.1	33.3	33.4	33.6
128-132	32.8	33.5	33.6	33.8	33.8	34.1	34.2	34.4	34.5
133-137	33.7	34.4	34.5	34.7	34.7	35.0	35.1	35.3	35.4
138-142	34.6	35.3	35.4	35.6	35.6	35.9	36.0	36.2	36.3
143-147	35.5	36.2	36.3	36.5	36.5	36.7	36.9	37.0	37.2
148-152	36.3	37.0	37.2	37.3	37.4	37.6	37.8	37.9	38.0
153-157	37.2	37.8	38.0	38.1	38.2	38.4	38.6	38.7	38.9
158-162	38.0	38.6	38.8	38.9	39.0	39.2	39.4	39.5	39.7
163-167	38.8	39.4	39.6	39.7	39.8	40.0	40.2	40.3	40.5
168-172	39.5	40.2	40.3	40.5	40.6	40.8	40.9	41.1	41.2
173-177	40.3	40.9	41.1	41.2	41.3	41.5	41.7	41.8	42.0
178-182	41.0	41.7	41.8	42.0	42.0	42.3	42.4	42.6	42.7
183-187	41.7	42.4	42.5	42.7	42.7	43.0	43.1	43.3	43.4
188-192	42.4	43.0	43.2	43.3	43.4	43.6	43.8	43.9	44.1
193-197	43.0	43.7	43.9	44.0	44.1	44.3	44.4	44.6	44.7
198-202	43.7	44.3	44.5	44.6	44.7	44.9	45.1	45.2	45.4

Table 4-6 Percent Fat Estimates for Three Sites—Men

Sum of 3 skinfolds	Age to last year								
	18-22	23-27	28-32	33-37	38-42	43-47	48-52	53-57	⩾ 58
8-12	1.8	2.6	3.4	4.2	4.9	5.7	6.5	7.3	8.1
13-17	3.6	4.4	5.2	6.0	6.8	7.6	8.4	9.1	9.9
18-22	5.4	6.2	7.0	7.8	8.6	9.3	10.1	10.9	11.7
23-27	7.1	7.9	8.7	9.5	10.3	11.1	11.9	12.6	13.4
28-32	8.8	9.6	10.4	11.2	12.0	12.8	13.5	14.3	15.1
33-37	10.4	11.2	12.0	12.8	13.6	14.4	15.2	15.9	16.7
38-42	12.0	12.8	13.6	14.4	15.2	15.9	16.7	17.5	18.3
43-47	13.5	14.3	15.1	15.9	16.7	17.5	18.3	19.0	19.8
48-52	15.0	15.8	16.6	17.4	18.1	18.9	19.7	20.5	21.3
53-57	16.4	17.2	18.0	18.8	19.6	20.3	21.1	21.9	22.7
58-62	17.8	18.5	19.3	20.1	20.9	21.7	22.5	23.3	24.1
63-67	19.1	19.9	20.6	21.4	22.2	23.0	23.8	24.6	25.4
68-72	20.3	21.1	21.9	22.7	23.5	24.3	25.1	25.8	26.6
73-77	21.5	22.3	23.1	23.9	24.7	25.5	26.3	27.0	27.8
78-82	22.7	23.5	24.3	25.0	25.8	26.6	27.4	28.2	29.0
83-87	23.8	24.6	25.3	26.1	26.9	27.7	28.5	29.3	30.1
88-92	24.8	25.6	26.4	27.2	28.0	28.8	29.6	30.3	31.1
93-97	25.8	26.6	27.4	28.2	29.0	29.8	30.5	31.3	32.1
98-102	26.7	27.5	28.3	29.1	29.9	30.7	31.5	32.3	33.1
103-107	27.6	28.4	29.2	30.0	30.8	31.6	32.4	33.2	33.9
108-112	28.5	29.3	30.1	30.8	31.6	32.4	33.2	34.0	34.8
113-117	29.3	30.0	30.8	31.6	32.4	33.2	34.0	34.8	35.6
118-122	30.0	30.8	31.6	32.4	33.1	33.9	34.7	35.5	36.3
123-127	30.7	31.5	32.2	33.0	33.8	34.6	35.4	36.2	37.0
128-132	31.3	32.1	32.9	33.7	34.4	35.2	36.0	36.8	37.6
133-137	31.9	32.7	33.4	34.2	35.0	35.8	36.6	37.4	38.2
138-142	32.4	33.2	34.0	34.8	35.5	36.3	37.1	37.9	38.7
143-147	32.9	33.6	34.4	35.2	36.0	36.8	37.6	38.4	39.2
148-152	33.3	34.1	34.8	35.6	36.4	37.2	38.0	38.8	39.6
153-157	33.6	34.4	35.2	36.0	36.8	37.6	38.4	39.2	39.9
158-162	33.9	34.7	35.5	36.3	37.1	37.9	38.7	39.5	40.3
163-167	34.2	35.0	35.8	36.6	37.4	38.1	38.9	39.7	40.5
168-172	34.4	35.2	36.0	36.8	37.6	38.4	39.1	39.9	40.7
173-177	34.6	35.3	36.1	36.9	37.7	38.5	39.3	40.1	40.9
178-182	34.7	35.4	36.2	37.0	37.8	38.6	39.4	40.2	41.0

Table 4-7 Percent Fat Estimates for Three Sites—Women

Sum of 3 skinfolds	Age to last year								
	18-22	23-27	28-32	33-37	38-42	43-47	48-52	53-57	⩾ 58
8-12	8.8	9.0	9.2	9.4	9.5	9.7	9.9	10.1	10.3
13-17	10.8	10.9	11.1	11.3	11.5	11.7	11.8	12.0	12.2
18-22	12.6	12.8	13.0	13.2	13.4	13.5	13.7	13.9	14.1
23-27	14.5	14.6	14.8	15.0	15.2	15.4	15.6	15.7	15.9
28-32	16.2	16.4	16.6	16.8	17.0	17.1	17.3	17.5	17.7
33-37	17.9	18.1	18.3	18.5	18.7	18.9	19.0	19.2	19.4
38-42	19.6	19.8	20.0	20.2	20.3	20.5	20.7	20.9	21.1
43-47	21.2	21.4	21.6	21.8	21.9	22.1	22.3	22.5	22.7
48-52	22.8	22.9	23.1	23.3	23.5	23.7	23.8	24.0	24.2
53-57	24.2	24.4	24.6	24.8	25.0	25.2	25.3	25.5	25.7
58-62	25.7	25.9	26.0	26.2	26.4	26.6	26.8	27.0	27.1
63-67	27.1	27.2	27.4	27.6	27.8	28.0	28.2	28.3	28.5
68-72	28.4	28.6	28.7	28.9	29.1	29.3	29.5	29.7	29.8
73-77	29.6	29.8	30.0	30.2	30.4	30.6	30.7	30.9	31.1
78-82	30.9	31.0	31.2	31.4	31.6	31.8	31.9	32.1	32.3
83-87	32.0	32.2	32.4	32.6	32.7	32.9	33.1	33.3	33.5
88-92	33.1	33.3	33.5	33.7	33.8	34.0	34.2	34.4	34.6
93-97	34.1	34.3	34.5	34.7	34.9	35.1	35.2	35.4	35.6
98-102	35.1	35.3	35.5	35.7	35.9	36.0	36.2	36.4	36.6
103-107	36.1	36.2	36.4	36.6	36.8	37.0	37.2	37.3	37.5
108-112	36.9	37.1	37.3	37.5	37.7	37.9	38.0	38.2	38.4
113-117	37.8	37.9	38.1	38.3	39.2	39.4	39.6	39.8	39.5
118-122	38.5	38.7	38.9	39.1	39.4	39.6	39.8	40.0	40.0
123-127	39.2	39.4	39.6	39.8	40.0	40.1	40.3	40.5	40.7
128-132	39.9	40.1	40.2	40.4	40.6	40.8	41.0	41.2	41.3
133-137	40.5	40.7	40.8	41.0	41.2	41.4	41.6	41.7	41.9
138-142	41.0	41.2	41.4	41.6	41.7	41.9	42.1	42.3	42.5
143-147	41.5	41.7	41.9	42.0	42.2	42.4	42.6	42.8	43.0
148-152	41.9	42.1	42.3	42.8	42.6	42.8	43.0	43.2	43.4
153-157	42.3	42.5	42.6	52.8	43.0	43.2	43.4	43.6	43.7
158-162	42.6	42.8	42.0	43.1	43.3	43.5	43.7	43.9	44.1
163-167	42.9	43.0	43.2	43.4	43.6	43.8	44.0	44.1	44.3
168-172	43.1	43.2	43.4	43.6	43.8	44.0	44.2	44.3	44.5
173-177	43.2	43.4	43.6	43.8	43.9	44.1	44.3	44.5	44.7
178-182	43.3	43.5	43.7	43.8	44.0	44.2	44.4	44.6	44.8

EXAMPLE 1: Subject A: male, 40 years old, 210 lb

Skinfold Measurements

Abdomen	31 mm
Ilium	26 mm
Tricep	14 mm
Thigh	21 mm
Sum of 4	92 mm

Using Table 4-4, which is the sum of four skinfolds for men, a total of 92 mm and an age of 40 at the last birthday yields a percentage of fat of 22.8. To find the target weight, turn to Table 4-2. Subject A has a target weight of 193 lb.

EXAMPLE 2: Subject B: female, 35 years old, 145 lb

Skinfold Measurements

Abdomen	28 mm
Ilium	23 mm
Tricep	18 mm
Thigh	33 mm
Sum of 4	102 mm

Using Table 4-5, which is the sum of four skinfolds for women, a total of 102 mm and an age of 35 at the last birthday yields a percentage of fat of 27.8. To find the target weight, turn to Table 4-3. Subject B has a target weight of 136 lb.

If the sum of four cannot be found because the thigh measurement cannot be taken, different charts must be used. The next two examples illustrate finding the target weight using three skinfold sites.

EXAMPLE 3: Subject A: male, 40 years old, 210 lb

Skinfold Measurements

Abdomen	31 mm
Ilium	26 mm
Tricep	14 mm
Sum of 3	71 mm

Using Table 4-6, which is the sum of three skinfolds for men, a total of 71 mm and an age of 40 at the last birthday yields a percentage of fat of 23.5. To find the target weight, turn to Table 4-2. Subject A has a target weight of 191 lb.

EXAMPLE 4: Subject B: female, 35 years old, 145 lb

Skinfold Measurements

Abdomen	28 mm
Ilium	23 mm
Tricep	18 mm
Sum of 3	69 mm

Using Table 4-7, which is the sum of three skinfolds for women, a total of 69 mm and an age of 35 at the last birthday yields a percentage of fat of 28.9. To find the target weight, turn to Table 4-3. Subject B has a target weight of 134 lb.

Skinfold Measurements

The skinfold measurements are used to determine the percent body fat as just described. The skinfold measurements as raw scores are also valuable and should supplement the information on percent body fat and target weight. Very often a participant in an exercise program reduces the subcutaneous fat in a number of locations, and these individual changes may not be identified in the estimation of percent fat alone. The skinfold measurement is an actual measurement and not a prediction and is therefore valuable in showing body-composition change. A more comprehensive evaluation can be made of the participant's progress if skinfolds are taken at several locations on the body. When these results are plotted on a norm scale, the changes that have occurred are visible and easily interpreted by the participant.

Descriptions of the location of skinfold measurements and the technique used in measuring are given next. *Although only three or four sites are used in the prediction of percent body fat, other sites are useful to measure for the skinfold profile.*

Test Administration

Skinfolds should be taken prior to active tests, as sweating and increased blood flow to the skin make measurement more difficult. Men can wear gym shorts for the test; women should wear shorts and a loose-fitting, sleeveless blouse or T-shirt that is also loose at the waist or the top to a two-piece swimsuit.

Equipment

1. A skinfold caliper (see Figs. 4-1 and 4-2) that conforms to specifications established by the committee of the Food and Nutrition Board of the National Research Council of the United States. The Lange and Harpenden calipers meet these specifications.
2. Testing forms to record data
3. Percent fat and target weight tables

Different types of calipers can produce considerably different measurements. The two types used by most YMCAs are the Lange (used by 65%) and the Harpenden (John Bull) (used by 33%). Two percent of YMCAs use some other type of caliper.

The standard pressure established for skinfold calipers is 10 g/mm² (10 grams of pressure for each square millimeter of caliper jaw surface). The Harpenden has a jaw surface of 90 mm² and the Lange 30 mm². This means that the Harpenden has a total pressure of 900 g and the Lange 580 g. The difference is supposedly accounted for by the distribution of pressure over the jaw surface, but the total pressure apparently does result in different measurements when calipers are compared.

Two current studies (Golding, 1988; Gruber & Pollock, 1988) are investigating these differences in calipers, and future research findings should be noted.

When Jackson and Pollock did the research that resulted in the prediction equations included in this book, they used Lange skinfold calipers; the tables and norms in this book thus are based on Lange measurements. As noted, 65% of the YMCAs reporting measurements for this book used Lange.

The difference in results between the Lange and the Harpenden calipers is not great (1 to 4 mm with a mean of 2.2) and does not result in big differences in final percentile ranks; however, when the sum of 4 is used for percent fat calculation, this small difference translates into 8.8 mm (2.2 × 4). Apparently the smaller the skinfold, the less difference in the measurements with different calipers.

Until further research is published it is suggested that those using Harpenden (John Bull) calipers add 2 mm to each skinfold site (8 for the sum of 4) prior to using the percent fat tables.

Procedure

Taking skinfolds requires practice to assure reliability and validity, as previously stated. The following suggestions for taking skinfold measurements should be observed: Take all measurements on the person's right side. Grasp the fold of skin firmly between the left thumb and four fingers, then lift it up. Pinch and lift the fold several times to be certain that no muscle is grasped. It requires a certain firmness to lift the skinfold accurately. Continue to hold the skinfold and place the contact surface of the calipers below the thumb and fingers. Do not let go of the fold. Release the grip on the caliper completely, allowing the spring to compress the fold. When the movement of the needle on the caliper dial stops, take the reading to the nearest half millimeter. (Note: The Harpenden caliper needle makes more than 1 revolution; the small pointer on the dial indicates the number of revolutions.) Keeping the left hand above the skinfold (see Figs. 4-3 through 4-16) allows the dial to be read easily. Remove the calipers, then release the fold.

It is important to measure skinfold accurately. Even after extensive practice, it is possible to make errors due to slight misplacement of the caliper or misreading of the dial. The following procedure is recommended:

a. The person measuring the skinfolds should not be the one recording them. An assistant should record the values as the measurer reads them from the caliper. It is helpful if the assistant repeats the values aloud as they are recorded.

b. Skinfolds should be lifted two or three times to determine the fold to be measured before placing the calipers. Too many individuals are overly anxious to put the calipers in place before determining what really should be measured.

c. Place the calipers below the thumb and four fingers and read the dial. Repeat this movement and again lift the fold two or three times, noting the reading on the caliper dial. Unless each measurement is close (1 to 2 mm), the readings will not be consistent, and reliability will be poor.

d. If several trials result in similar measurements, record the last measurement.

e. Do not lift the skinfold on the actual measurement site, as the calipers will be too far forward. The jaws of the caliper must be on the exact site. Adjust finger grip as necessary.

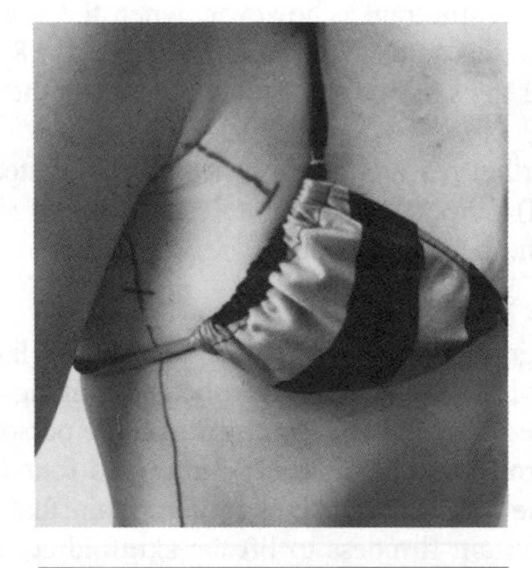

Figure 4-3. Location of pectoral skinfold.

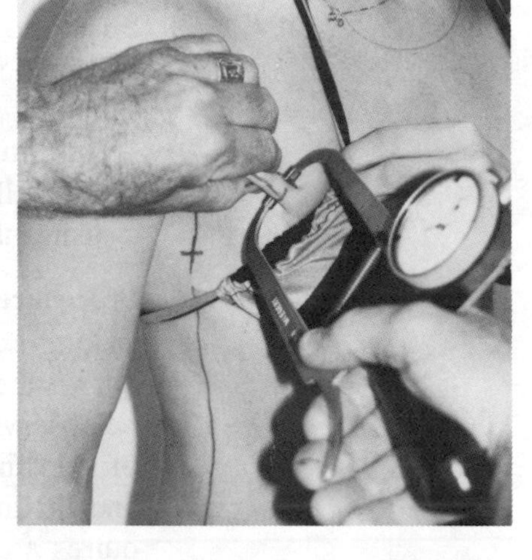

Figure 4-4. Measurement of pectoral skinfold.

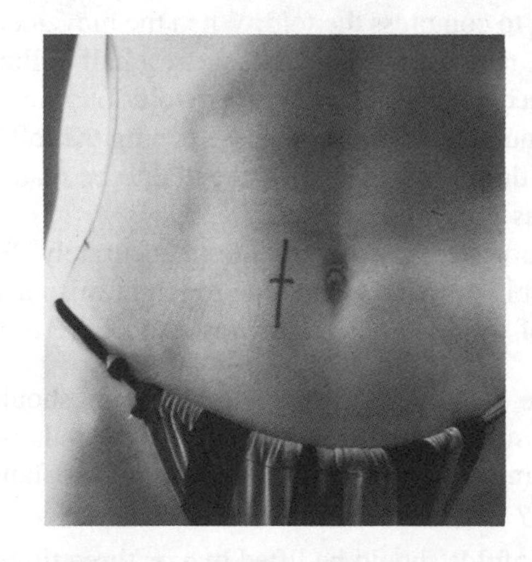

Figure 4-5. Location of abdominal skinfold.

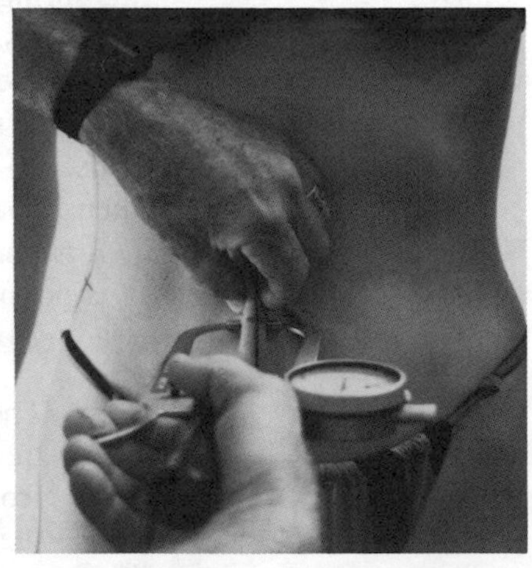

Figure 4-6. Measurement of abdominal skinfold.

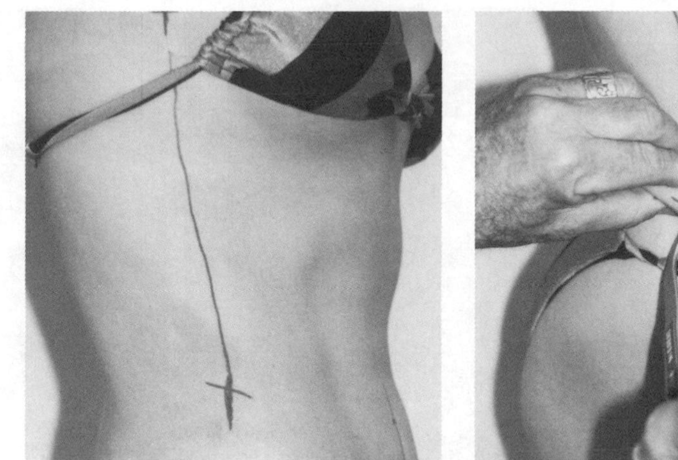

Figure 4-7. Location of hip skinfold.

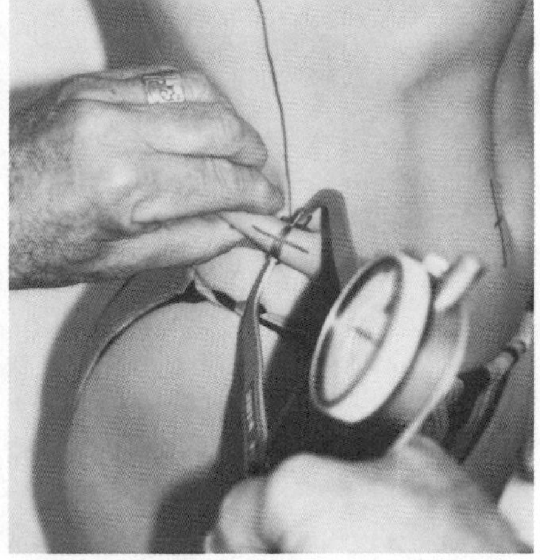

Figure 4-8. Measurement of hip skinfold.

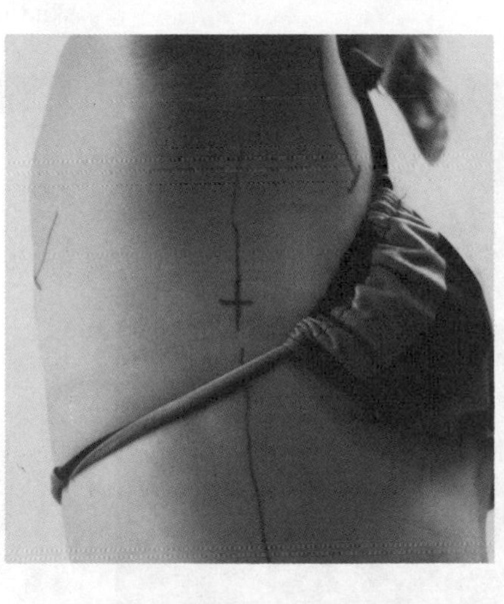

Figure 4-9. Location of axilla skinfold.

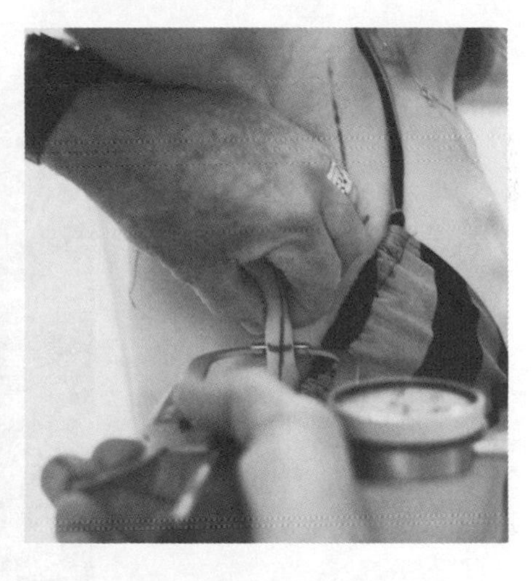

Figure 4-10. Measurement of axilla skinfold.

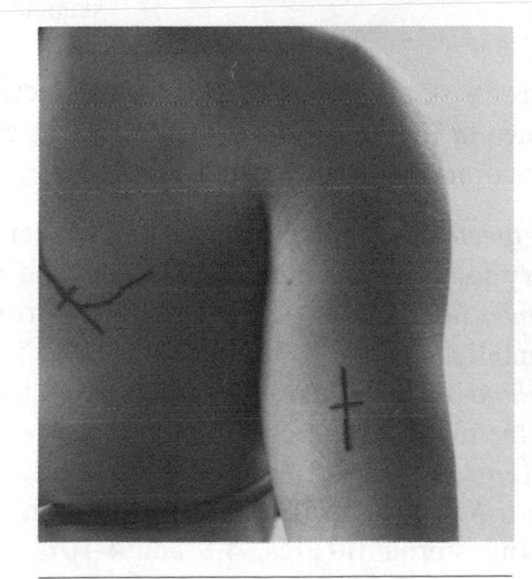

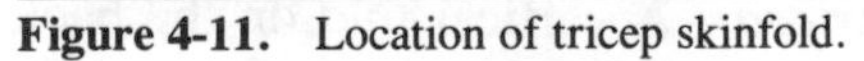

Figure 4-11. Location of tricep skinfold.

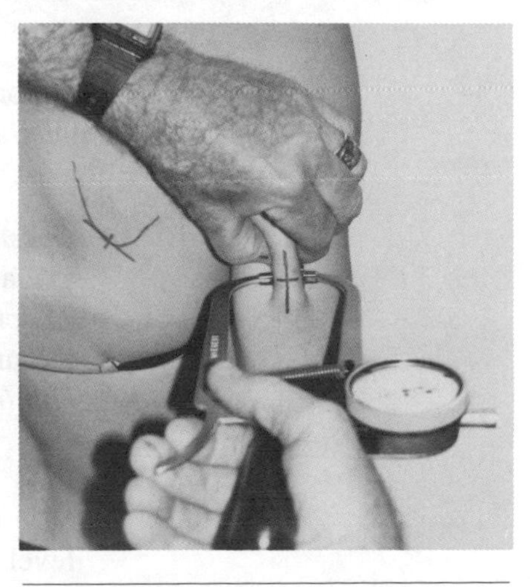

Figure 4-12. Measurement of tricep skinfold.

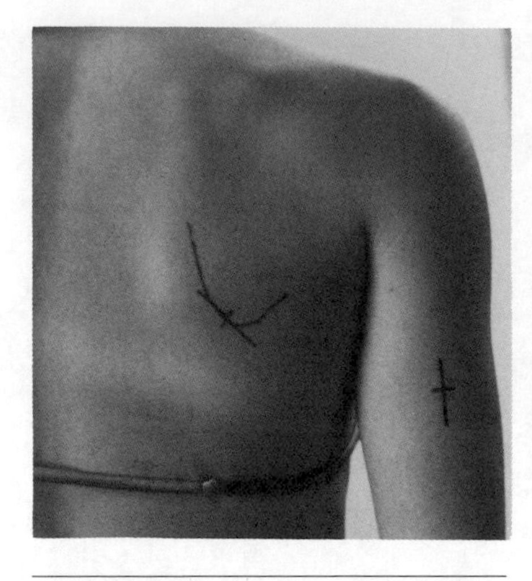

Figure 4-13. Location of scapula skinfold.

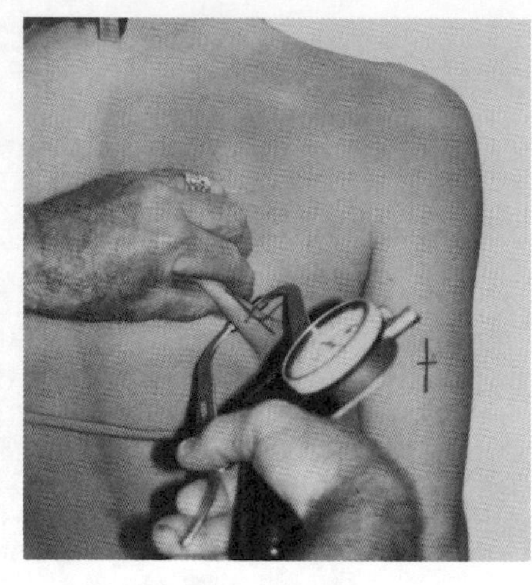

Figure 4-14. Measurement of scapula skinfold.

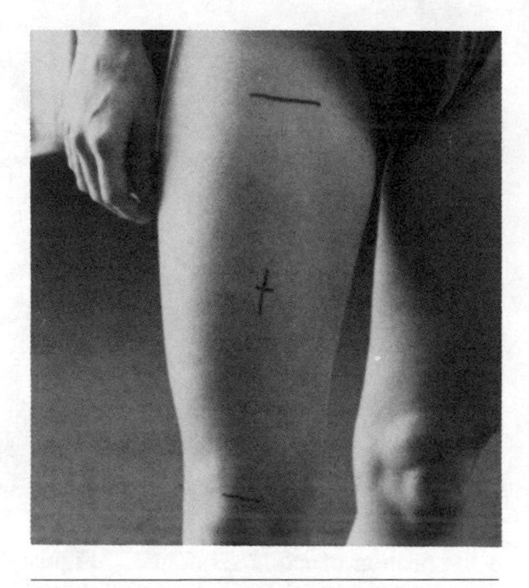

Figure 4-15. Location of thigh skinfold.

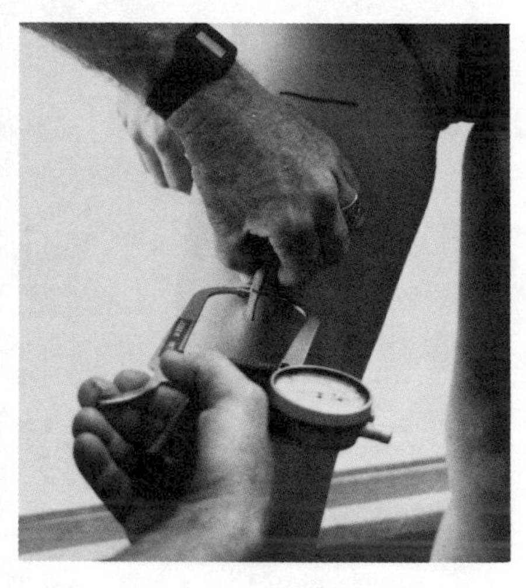

Figure 4-16. Measurement of thigh skinfold.

Locations for skinfold measurements are described in the following text and are illustrated in Figures 4-3 through 4-16. The sites are where measurements are taken and are not grip locations.

- *Chest (pectoral).* A diagonal fold on the pectoral line midway between the axillary fold and the nipple (Figs. 4-3 and 4-4)
- *Abdomen (umbilicus).* A vertical fold approximately 1 in. to the right of the umbilicus (Figs. 4-5 and 4-6)
- *Hip (ilium or suprailium).* A diagonal fold just above the crest of the ilium (i.e., the highest peak on the side of the pelvic girdle on the midaxillary line) (Figs. 4-7 and 4-8)
- *Side (axilla, midaxilla).* A vertical fold on the midaxillary line at nipple level (midsternum) (Figs. 4-9 and 4-10)
- *Arm (tricep).* A vertical fold on the back of the upper arm midway between the shoulder and elbow joints (Figs. 4-11 and 4-12)
- *Back (scapula, subscapula).* A diagonal fold or the inferior angle of the scapula (Figs. 4-13 and 4-14)

- *Thigh (leg).* A vertical fold on the front of the thigh midway between groin line and the top of the patella (Figs. 4-15 and 4-16)

Results can be compared to the norm scales on the Body Composition Profile forms at the end of this chapter. If Harpenden calipers are used, make the correction before determining percent fat. The YMCA norms are developed for the seven sites described earlier. Other sites can be used; however, YMCA norms will not be applicable. Norms for those particular sites will need to be obtained.

Cardiorespiratory Evaluation

The bicycle ergometer test has been selected for individual cardiorespiratory fitness evaluation. It is used with the understanding that the participant has been examined by his or her personal physician and has received clearance to participate in YMCA fitness testing and subsequent exercise programs.

The bicycle test, which predicts maximum working capacity by measuring the response to submaximal work, can also be used as a means of predicting maximum oxygen consumption. Although the latter is an additional measurement that can be determined from the results of this test, it is not the primary purpose of the bicycle test presented here.

A step test also is available for use in group testing. It is an excellent substitute for the bicycle ergometer test when there is not enough equipment or staff to administer individual tests.

It is desirable for participants in their first year of fitness training to repeat testing once after about 10 to 12 weeks and then again at the end of 6 to 12 months. This will show participants their personal responses to training and will possibly act as a motivator for continued participation. After the first year of exercise in the fitness program, most individuals need not be tested more than once a year.

The measurements resulting from the bicycle test or the step test reflect the cardiorespiratory response of the individual and should be used to show changes in endurance during the exercise training program. If an individual scores in either the *fair* or *poor* categories of either the bicycle test or the step test (see Physical Fitness Evaluation Profile for rating scales), he or she should start out more slowly in the exercise program than should those scoring *average* or above. These individuals may not have the cardiorespiratory capacity to perform moderate to strenuous work and may start out with a walking program for several weeks before beginning the exercise class. In any case, signs of overexertion should be watched for during the first few weeks of the program. Individuals who score in the *average*, *good*, or *excellent* categories should be able to start out in the regular beginner's program and can handle an exercise program commensurate with their fitness rating.

Physical Working Capacity Test

In recent years, especially since the advent of the Y's Way to Physical Fitness, there has been an increased utilization of bicycle ergometers in YMCAs and physical fitness laboratories. The bicycle ergometer offers several advantages over a treadmill:

- Less expensive
- Requires little space

- Easily transported
- Easier to take heart rate
- Requires little or no training or practice
- External work is known

The most commonly used tests on the bicycle include the PWC 170 as developed by Sjostrand (1947) and the estimation of maximal oxygen uptake by Åstrand and Rhyming (1954). Both tests are based on the fact that heart rate and oxygen uptake are linear functions of the rate of work. In the Åstrand and Rhyming test the purpose is to estimate the individual's maximal oxygen uptake, which is highly related to the individual's capacity for heavy, prolonged work.

There is a linear relationship between heart rate (HR) and work (W); however, this linearity exists only at certain heart rates. At low heart rates, many external stimuli can affect the heart rate (e.g., talking, laughter, and nervousness). However, once the heart starts pumping harder as the muscles demand more blood, external stimuli no longer affect the heart rate, and linearity occurs at about 110 bpm. The relationship between heart rate and work increases in a linear fashion until it plateaus, signaling the maximum heart rate. A 70-year-old man will plateau at about 150, and, as 70-year-olds will usually be the oldest individuals tested on the bicycle, almost everyone will be linear between 110 and 150 bpm (see Fig. 4-17).

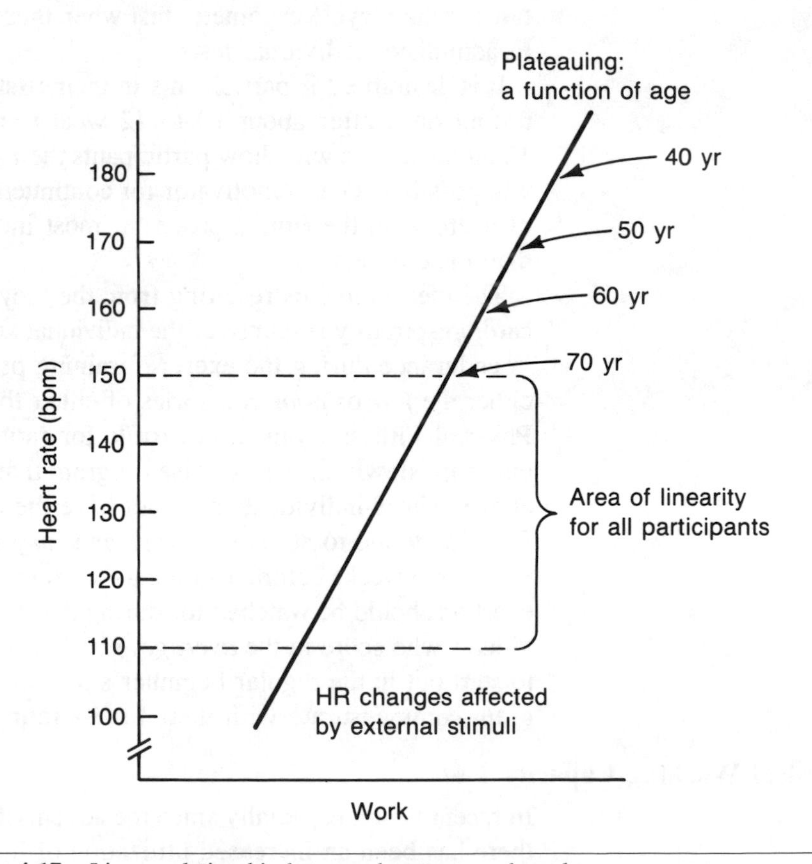

Figure 4-17. Linear relationship between heart rate and work.

The basis of this test is to establish the linearity between heart rate and work for the person being tested. To establish a line, two points are needed; therefore two workloads are used. The only precaution is that these two points must be in the linear portion of the relationship. The workloads cannot be too high or too low.

Linearity begins at approximately 110 bpm. The plateauing due to reaching maximum heart rate is a function of age; however, at a heart rate of 150 bpm, almost everyone tested will still be linear. Therefore, linearity is said to be between 110 and 150 bpm.

To eliminate the need to guess the workload required to start the test, a guide to setting workloads is presented in Figure 4-18. By using this table a tester should be able to eliminate the possibility of presenting too difficult a workload for the participant. The workload chart should be used conservatively, as it is better to give too small than too large a workload.

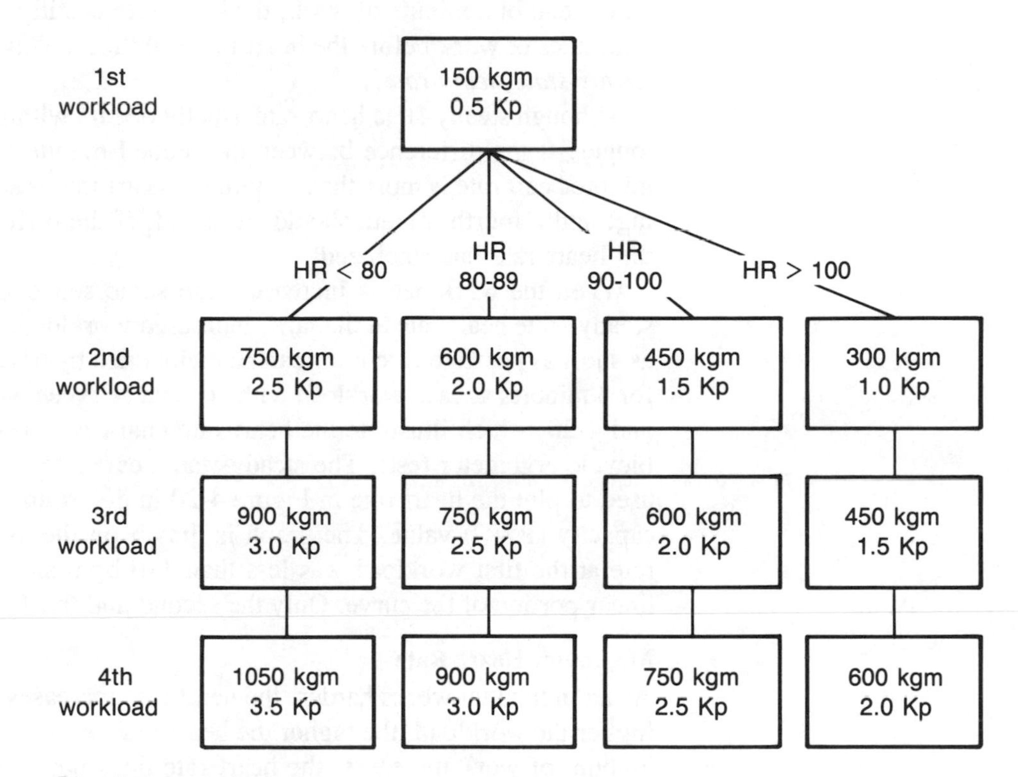

Directions:

1. Set the first workload at 150 kgm/min (0.5 Kp).
2. If the HR in the third min is
   - less than (<) 80, set the second load at 750 kgm (2.5 Kp);
   - 80 to 89, set the second load at 600 kgm (2.0 Kp);
   - 90 to 100, set the second load at 450 kgm (1.5 Kp);
   - greater than (>) 100, set the second load at 300 kgm (1.0 Kp).
3. Set the third and fourth (if required) loads according to the loads in the columns below the second loads.

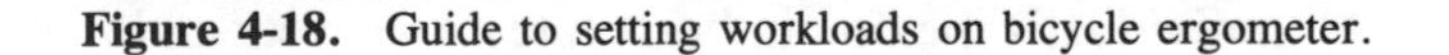

Figure 4-18. Guide to setting workloads on bicycle ergometer.

The first workload is given to determine the heart-rate response elicited for a small workload. Usually this first workload will not be plotted because the heart rate will be under 110 bpm; however, should the heart rate be above 110 bpm, it should be used. Then only one more workload will be necessary to plot the line. If the heart rate is not 110 bpm or greater, then two more workloads will be needed to plot points.

Many laboratories doing research use three plot points. Because these three points will seldom be on an exact line, a line of best fit must be computed. There is no significant difference between using two points or three or more points.

As part of understanding the bicycle test, the concepts of *steady-state heart rate, maximum heart rate*, and *maximum oxygen uptake* should be understood.

Steady-State Heart Rate

The moment a participant starts to work, the heart rate immediately increases. At the end of a minute of work, the heart rate is still increasing. It takes about 3 minutes of work before the heart rate stabilizes. This plateauing is called the *steady-state heart rate*.

Although steady-state heart rate usually occurs within 3 minutes, it may take longer. If the difference between the second-minute heart rate and the third-minute heart rate is more than 5 bpm, the heart rate is still significantly increasing, and a fourth minute should be added. If the difference is 5 or less bpm, the heart rate has stabilized.

When the workload is increased, the same sequence occurs to establish a steady-state heart rate at the new, increased workload. As the test is to be kept as short as possible, accuracy can be maintained by having the participant pedal for 3 minutes at each workload with no rests between workloads (see Figs. 4-19 and 4-20, which illustrate the heart-rate changes in response to a progressive bicycle ergometer test). The steady-state heart rate (SSHR) in Figure 4-19 is used to plot the heart rate in Figure 4-20 in determining the physical working capacity (PWC) value. The graph is drawn on the assumption that the heart rate at the first workload was less than 110 bpm and therefore is outside the linear portion of the curve. Only the second and third workloads were plotted.

Maximum Heart Rate

As an individual works harder, the heart rate increases in a linear fashion. The higher the workload, the higher the heart rate. At some point, even though the amount of work increases, the heart rate does not increase. At this point the heart has reached its fastest rate or *maximum heart rate*. Everyone has a point at which the heart rate will go no higher, although this point differs among individuals due to various reasons. The main reason is age. As one ages, the ability to drive the heart to high rates decreases. This decrease in maximum heart rate is partly due to a decrease in physical fitness, and in the general population this decrease is very evident. However, in fit individuals who continue aerobic activity into later life this decrease is not so rapid.

It has been shown that maximum heart rate decreases with age in a linear fashion as depicted in Figure 4-17. The formula of 220 minus age predicts an individual's maximum heart rate. A 40-year-old male would have a predicted maximum heart rate of 180. This prediction is only representative of the average for a population of 40-year-old males and does not take into account individual variations.

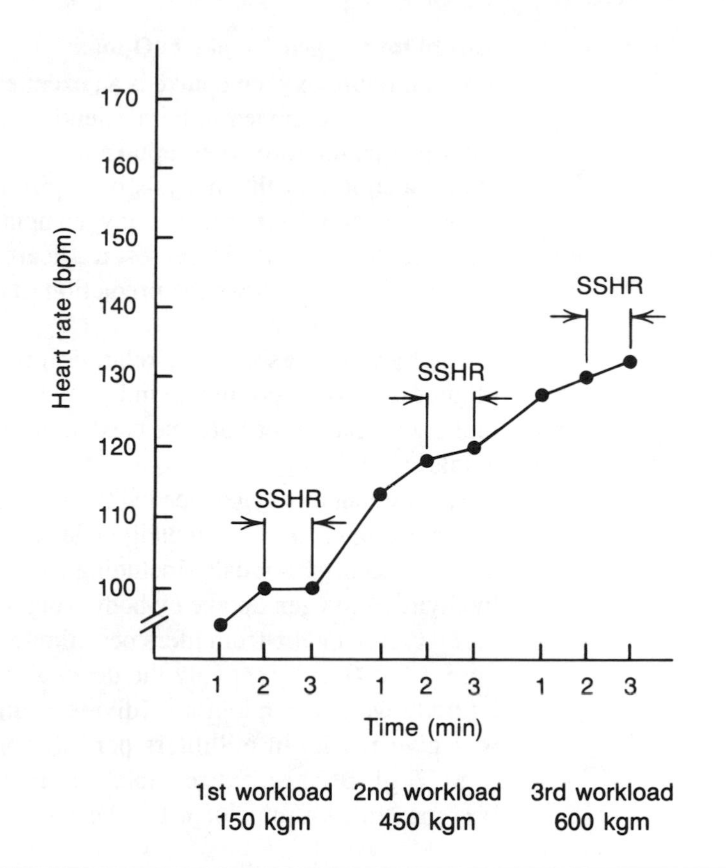

Figure 4-19. Example of heart-rate changes during bicycle ergometer test.

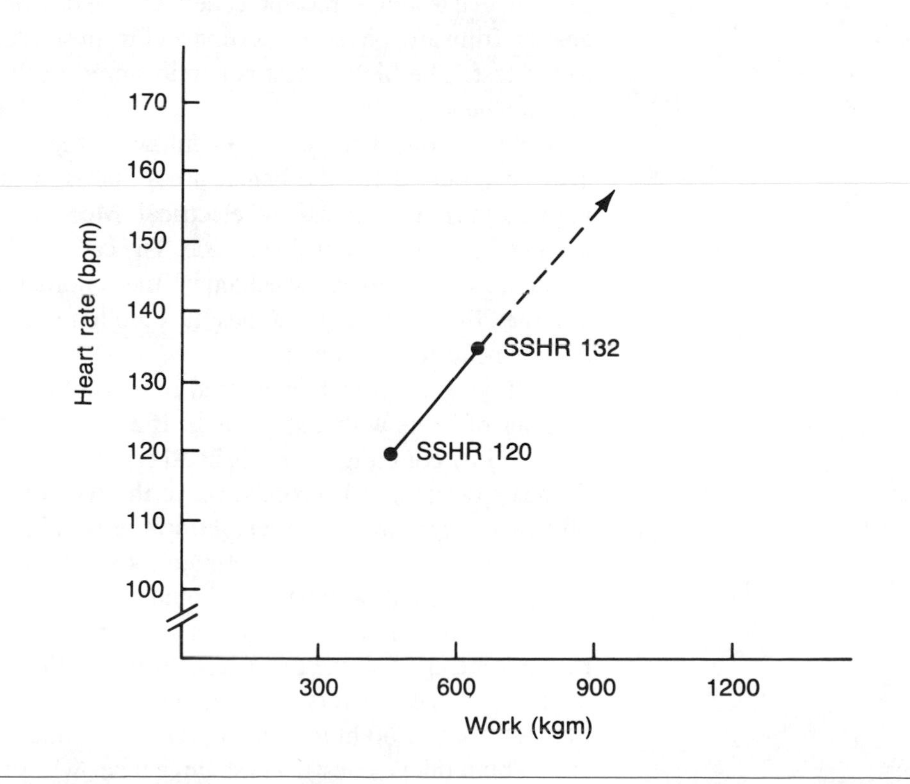

Figure 4-20. Example of plotting steady-state heart rate to determine physical working capacity.

Maximum Oxygen Uptake ($\dot{V}O_2max$)

The maximum oxygen uptake is an excellent test of cardiorespiratory efficiency and is often mentioned in both scientific and popular literature. The measurement of maximum oxygen uptake is a laboratory technique that involves both the collection and the analysis of expired air during exercise; however, it is known that both heart rate and oxygen uptake have a linear relationship to workload. As the workload increases, the heart rate and the oxygen uptake increase. This relationship allows the prediction of a maximum oxygen uptake from the maximum heart rate.

The bicycle test shows the relationship of heart rate to work and thereby can predict the workload that an individual would be capable of handling at maximum heart rate. It can also be used to predict an individual's maximum oxygen uptake.

The amount of oxygen needed for any task is a function of size (i.e., weight), so oxygen uptakes between individuals can be compared only if weight is equalized between individuals, including males and females. This is accomplished by dividing oxygen uptake by body weight. (Note: For ease of calculation, convert oxygen uptake from liters per minute to milliliters per minute by multiplying by 1,000 or by moving the decimal point three places to the right; divide by body weight in kilograms [divide pounds by 2.2 to get kilograms] and this will give results in milliliters per kilogram [milliliters divided by kilograms = mL/kg]. Because oxygen uptake is always given per minute, this expression becomes mL/kg/min, or $mL \cdot kg^{-1} \cdot min^{-1}$. See Table 4-10.)

Test Administration

Because some individuals are unfamiliar with bicycling, a practice session prior to the actual testing is recommended. On the day of testing, the participant should abstain from any physical exertion and from smoking or eating for 2 hours prior to the test. The bicycle test is administered in the same manner for both men and women.

A metronome is required to administer the bicycle ergometer test and will also be required for the bench press and step tests. There are two kinds of metronomes: mechanical and electrical. Mechanical metronomes typically have a wand that moves from side to side. The cadence is changed by moving a weight up or down the wand. Mechanical metronomes must be manually wound to operate. Electrical metronomes have both an auditory and a visual signal and do not need to be wound.

Both types of metronomes need to be calibrated. This is done by timing the number of beats with a stopwatch. If a metronome is set for 100 bpm, it may be tested by counting the beats in 30 seconds and multiplying by 2. If less than 50 beats occur in 30 seconds, move the weight down the wand; if more than 50 beats occur, move the weight up the wand. Time the beats again, making adjustments until the cadence matches the time.

Metronomes usually have no volume control and are often too quiet for testing. One answer to this problem is to make an audio tape recording of the metronome and use the recording during testing sessions. This allows volume control and makes a very efficient metronome. Three 60-minute tapes are recommended: one at 60 bpm (bench press test), one at 96 bpm (step test), and one at 100 bpm (bicycle test). These three tapes will supply all the metronome needs for the test battery and will eliminate any need for future calibration.

Equipment

1. An accurate, easily calibrated, constant torque bicycle ergometer with a range of 0 to 2,100 kilogram-meters (kgm) per minute (see Fig. 4-21). A kilogram-meter is a unit of work that is equal to the energy required to lift 1 kg (2.2 lb) vertically a distance of 1 m (3.3 ft). Each major gradation should be at 300 kgm, with intermediate marks at 150 kgm. As the Monark bicycle ergometer is the one most commonly used in YMCAs, it is used in the examples; other brands meeting these criteria may be used.
2. A metronome set at 100 bpm.
3. A timer to time riding duration.
4. A stopwatch to time heart rate.
5. A stethoscope to count heart rate.
6. Testing forms to record data.

Note: No recovery HRs are used in the bicycle ergometer test.

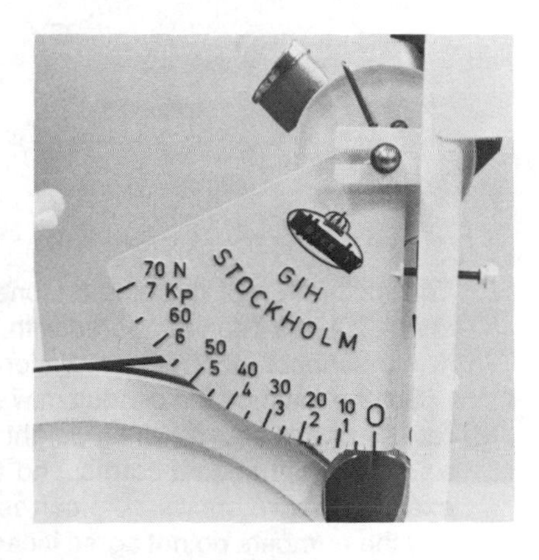

Figure 4-21. Workload scale on bicycle ergometer.

Procedure

Check the calibration of the bicycle. On the Monark be sure the red line on the pendulum weight reads 0 on the workload scale before starting. Moving an adjusting wing nut easily corrects this if it is not in line (see Fig. 4-22 on how to calibrate the bicycle). If another brand of bicycle ergometer is used, follow the manufacturer's instructions for calibration. As there is a slight difference in resistance between bicycles, be sure that any retesting is done on the same bicycle.

Briefly explain the concept of the test to the participant and fill out the test forms.

Adjust the seat height on the ergometer. When the pedal is at its lowest point the knee should be straight, with the ball of the foot on the pedal and the leg stretched. Note the seat position on the score sheet so that it may be used in retesting.

Set the metronome at either 50 or 100 bpm and allow the participant to pedal freewheel (no load) for a minute to get the pace. At 50 revolutions per minute

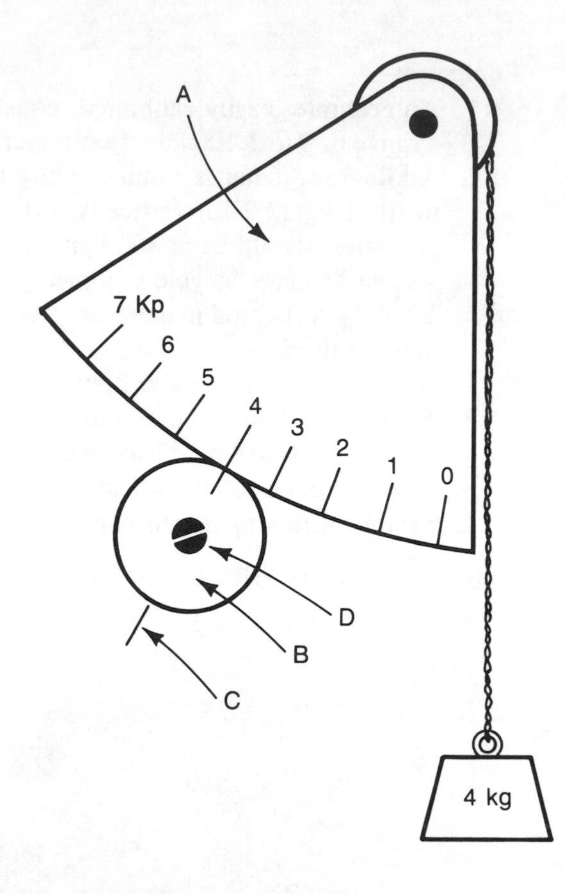

The calibration of the bike is done precisely at the factory and unless the adjusting screw (C) has been tampered with, seldom is there a need for recalibration. However, if you suspect incorrect calibration it can be checked as follows.

Set the mark on the pendulum weight (B) at 0. Attach a weight known to be very accurate as shown above. A 1 kg weight should correspond to a reading of 1 on the scale (A); a 2 kg weight should correspond to a reading of 2 on the scale (A); and so on. The example above shows 4 kg corresponding to 4 on the scale.

If the numbers do not agree it can be corrected by changing the adjusting screw (C). This screw moves the center of gravity of the pendulum (this screw is locked with the screw D).

Figure 4-22. Bicycle ergometer calibration. *Note.* From *Work Tests With the Bicycle Ergometer* (p. 14) by P.-O. Åstrand, n.d., Varberg, Sweden: Monark. Copyright by Monark-Crescent AB. Adapted by permission.

(rpm) the right foot makes 50 complete revolutions in one minute. The metronome set at 100 bpm means that at each "click" a foot (left or right) should be on the downstroke. This is still 50 rpm.

Set the initial workload at 150 kgm/min (see Fig. 4-18 for workload guidelines). On the Monark ergometer, one complete turn of the pedals on the bicycle moves the wheel 6 m. At a pedaling rate of 50 rpm, the total distance covered in 1 minute is 300 m. If the scale is set so that 1 kg of force is acting on the wheel, then 300 m/min • 1 kg = 300 kgm/min. Table 4-8 gives the workload in kgm/min for each scale setting on the Monark bicycle ergometer.

Allow the participant to work at the first workload for 3 minutes. Count the heart rate at the second and third minutes (see Fig. 4-23). The difference in heart rates between the second and third minutes should not vary by more than

Table 4-8 Scale Setting and Workload on Bicycle Ergometer

Scale setting	Workload (kgm/min)	Scale setting	Workload (kgm/min)
.5 Kp	150	4.5 Kp	1350
1.0 Kp	300	5.0 Kp	1500
1.5 Kp	450	5.5 Kp	1650
2.0 Kp	600	6.0 Kp	1800
2.5 Kp	750	6.5 Kp	1950
3.0 Kp	900	7.0 Kp	2100
3.5 Kp	1050		
4.0 Kp	1200		

five beats; if it does, extend the ride for an extra minute or until a stable value is obtained. Take the time for 30 beats. Start the stopwatch on a beat, counting it as "zero," and stop the watch at 30 beats. See the heart-rate conversion chart (Table 4-9) to find beats per minute. Check the steady-state heart rate against Figure 4-18 as a guide to setting the workloads. Remember that the purpose of this guide is to set the task in small increments so that the workload does not cause the heart rate to increase too rapidly or to reach too high a level. Conservatism is the rule. An extra workload will not change the test, and the test should be submaximal, so keep it that way. Record the heart rate carefully.

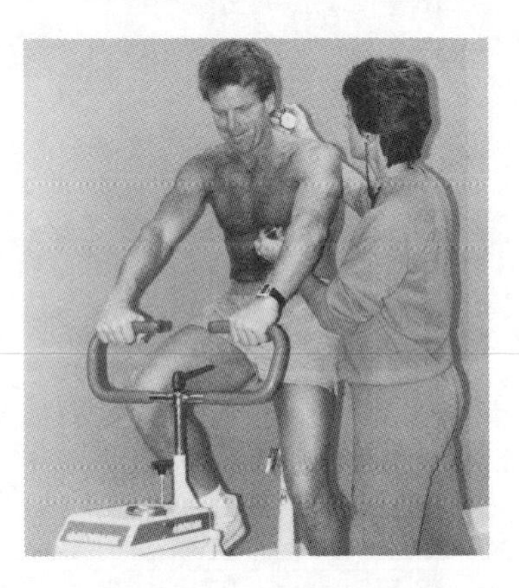

Figure 4-23. Taking heart rate on bicycle ergometer.

Change the workload. There is no need to hurry to change it, as the participant may ride 4 or 5 minutes at each workload. Take time to record the heart rate properly after each workload before putting in the next workload. Reset the clock and record the new workload on the score sheet. As each participant's second and third workloads will differ, enter these on the score sheet as soon as they are determined to avoid errors later.

Regularly check the workload setting during each workload period. As the friction belt gets hot, it may slip, giving less resistance. Returning it to the desired workload will ensure that the participant is doing the workload that is required.

As the steady-state heart rate is being elicited at each workload, it is not critical exactly when the heart rate is taken. For consistency the heart rate should

Table 4-9 Heart-Rate Conversion Chart (30 beats to bpm)

Sec	bpm	Sec	bpm	Sec	bpm
22.0	82	17.3	104	12.6	143
21.9	82	17.2	105	12.5	144
21.8	83	17.1	105	12.4	145
21.7	83	17.0	106	12.3	146
21.6	83	16.9	107	12.2	148
21.5	84	16.8	107	12.1	149
21.4	84	16.7	108	12.0	150
21.3	85	16.6	108	11.9	151
21.2	85	16.5	109	11.8	153
21.1	85	16.4	110	11.7	154
21.0	86	16.3	110	11.6	155
20.9	86	16.2	111	11.5	157
20.8	87	16.1	112	11.4	158
20.7	87	16.0	113	11.3	159
20.6	87	15.9	113	11.2	161
20.5	88	15.8	114	11.1	162
20.4	88	15.7	115	11.0	164
20.3	89	15.6	115	10.9	165
20.2	89	15.5	116	10.8	167
20.1	90	15.4	117	10.7	168
20.0	90	15.3	118	10.6	170
19.9	90	15.2	118	10.5	171
19.8	91	15.1	119	10.4	173
19.7	91	15.0	120	10.3	175
19.6	92	14.9	121	10.2	176
19.5	92	14.8	122	10.1	178
19.4	93	14.7	122	10.0	180
19.3	93	14.6	123	9.9	182
19.2	94	14.5	124	9.8	184
19.1	94	14.4	125	9.7	186
19.0	95	14.3	126	9.6	188
18.9	95	14.2	127	9.5	189
18.8	96	14.1	128	9.4	191
18.7	96	14.0	129	9.3	194
18.6	97	13.9	129	9.2	196
18.5	97	13.8	130	9.1	198
18.4	98	13.7	131	9.0	200
18.3	98	13.6	132	8.9	202
18.2	99	13.5	133	8.8	205
18.1	99	13.4	134	8.7	207
18.0	100	13.3	135	8.6	209
17.9	101	13.2	136	8.5	212
17.8	101	13.1	137	8.4	214
17.7	102	13.0	138	8.3	217
17.6	102	12.9	140	8.2	220
17.5	103	12.8	141	8.1	222
17.4	103	12.7	142	8.0	225

Note. From *Work Tests With the Bicycle Ergometer* (p. 17) by P.-O. Åstrand, n.d., Varberg, Sweden: Monark. Copyright by Monark-Crescent AB. Reprinted by permission.

be taken as the full 2- and 3-minute marks are reached. This means that the participant actually rides a little longer than 3 minutes.

After the second workload is completed, record the heart rate at the end of the second and third minutes. Again, these should not differ by more than five beats. Unless the first workload produces a heart rate of 110 bpm or more, determine the third workload and proceed. If the first workload did produce 110 bpm, there is no need for a third workload.

Throughout the test watch for exertional intolerance or other signs of undue fatigue or unusual response. Instruct the participant to indicate how he or she feels from time to time. Do not engage the participant in conversation during the testing.

Record the heart rate at the end of the second and third minutes of the third workload. The test is now complete. Allow the participant to cool down by riding at no resistance.

Scoring

Once the test is complete, the final heart rate in each of the workloads to be used (the two between 110 bpm and 150 bpm) should be plotted against the respective workload on Figure 4-24. The first load is not used in this calculation unless it exceeded 110 bpm. A straight line is drawn through the two points and extended to that participant's predicted maximal heart rate.

The point at which the diagonal line intersects the horizontal predicted maximal heart-rate line represents the maximal working capacity for that participant. A perpendicular line should be dropped from this point to the baseline where the maximal physical workload capacity can be read in kgm/min.

EXAMPLES: Plotting the Maximal Physical Working Capacity

The first subject has been given all three workloads according to the previously described directions. The results follow.

Age _40_ years Weight _176_ lb _80_ kg

PHYSICAL WORKING CAPACITY TEST

Seat Height _8_ Predicted Max Heart Rate _180_ bpm

85% of Predicted Max Heart Rate _153_ bpm _11.8_ Seconds for 30 Beats

WORKLOADS		HEART RATES	
1st Workload	150 kgm	101	2nd min
		105	3rd min
		______	4th min (if needed)
2nd Workload	300 kgm	116	2nd min
		120	3rd min
		______	4th min (if needed)
3rd Workload	450 kgm	145	2nd min
		145	3rd min
		______	4th min (if needed)

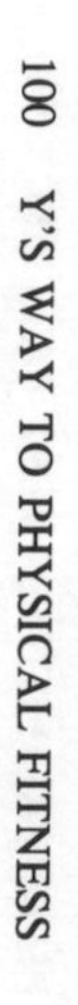

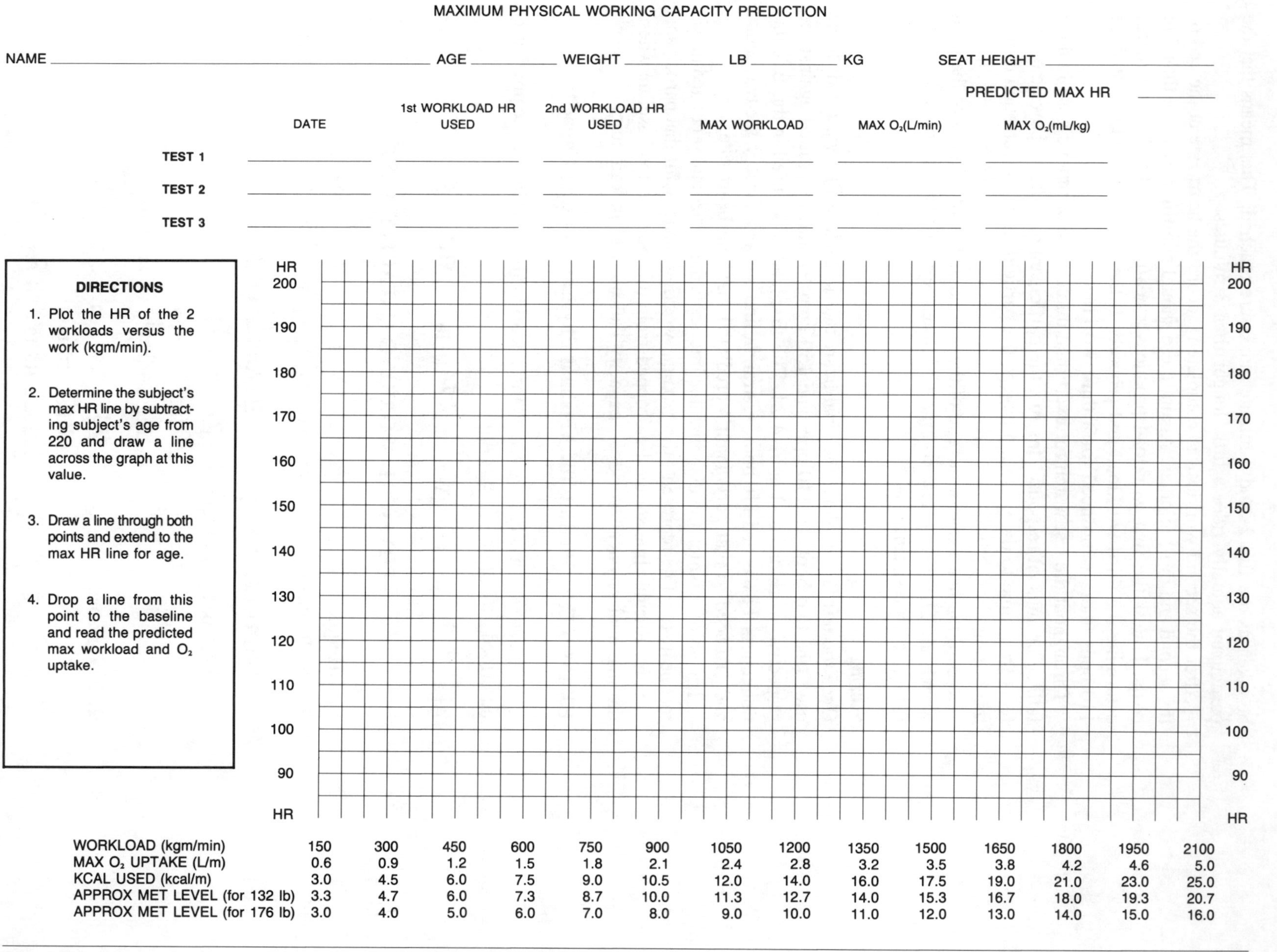

MAXIMUM PHYSICAL WORKING CAPACITY PREDICTION

NAME ______ AGE ______ WEIGHT ______ LB ______ KG ______ SEAT HEIGHT ______

PREDICTED MAX HR ______

	DATE	1st WORKLOAD HR USED	2nd WORKLOAD HR USED	MAX WORKLOAD	MAX O_2(L/min)	MAX O_2(mL/kg)
TEST 1						
TEST 2						
TEST 3						

DIRECTIONS

1. Plot the HR of the 2 workloads versus the work (kgm/min).
2. Determine the subject's max HR line by subtracting subject's age from 220 and draw a line across the graph at this value.
3. Draw a line through both points and extend to the max HR line for age.
4. Drop a line from this point to the baseline and read the predicted max workload and O_2 uptake.

WORKLOAD (kgm/min)	150	300	450	600	750	900	1050	1200	1350	1500	1650	1800	1950	2100
MAX O_2 UPTAKE (L/m)	0.6	0.9	1.2	1.5	1.8	2.1	2.4	2.8	3.2	3.5	3.8	4.2	4.6	5.0
KCAL USED (kcal/m)	3.0	4.5	6.0	7.5	9.0	10.5	12.0	14.0	16.0	17.5	19.0	21.0	23.0	25.0
APPROX MET LEVEL (for 132 lb)	3.3	4.7	6.0	7.3	8.7	10.0	11.3	12.7	14.0	15.3	16.7	18.0	19.3	20.7
APPROX MET LEVEL (for 176 lb)	3.0	4.0	5.0	6.0	7.0	8.0	9.0	10.0	11.0	12.0	13.0	14.0	15.0	16.0

Figure 4-24. Form for plotting maximum physical working capacity prediction.

The heart rates in the third minute of the second and third workloads are plotted against their respective workloads. This entire calculation is shown in Figure 4-25. A line is drawn through these points and extended to the predicted maximum heart rate line as determined by age (i.e., 220 − 40 = 180). A line is dropped to the baseline at the intersection of these two lines, and the predicted maximum workload is determined (i.e., 650 kgm/min). Maximum oxygen uptake can also be predicted from this test. The predicted maximum oxygen uptake in this example is 1.6 L/m, or 1,600 mL. Divided by body weight in kilograms this would compute to a maximum oxygen uptake in mL/kg ($\dot{V}O_2max$) of 20 mL of oxygen for every kilogram of body weight in 1 minute, written as mL/kg/min. This is written in the scientific literature as $mL \cdot kg^{-1} \cdot min^{-1}$. This calculation is made easy by the use of Table 4-10. Enter weight and maximum $\dot{V}O_2$, and where the two intersect is the mL/kg/min value.

A second subject has been given only two workloads because the first workload elicited a heart rate greater than 110 bpm. The test was given according to the previously described directions. Here are the results.

Age __30__ years Weight __121__ lb __55__ kg

PHYSICAL WORKING CAPACITY TEST

Seat Height __6__ Predicted Max Heart Rate __190__ bpm

85% of Predicted Max Heart Rate __161__ bpm __11.2__ Seconds for 30 Beats

WORKLOADS		**HEART RATES**	
1st Workload	150 kgm	110	2nd min
		112	3rd min
		______	4th min (if needed)
2nd Workload	300 kgm	124	2nd min
		125	3rd min
		______	4th min (if needed)

3rd workload not necessary

The heart rate in the final minute of the first and second workloads is plotted against the respective workloads. This entire calculation is shown in Figure 4-26.

A line is drawn through these points and extended to the predicted maximum heart-rate line. Where the lines intersect, a perpendicular line is dropped to the baseline. This indicates a predicted PWC maximum of 1,050 kgm/min for this example. This means that, had the subject been worked until the maximum heart rate was elicited, he or she would have been cycling at 1,050 kgm. The predicted maximum oxygen uptake is 2.4 L/min. Divided by body weight in kilograms this would give a maximum oxygen uptake of 43.64 mL/kg/min ($\dot{V}O_2$ divided by weight, or 2,400 mL ÷ 55 kg). This calculation is made easy by the use of Table 4-10.

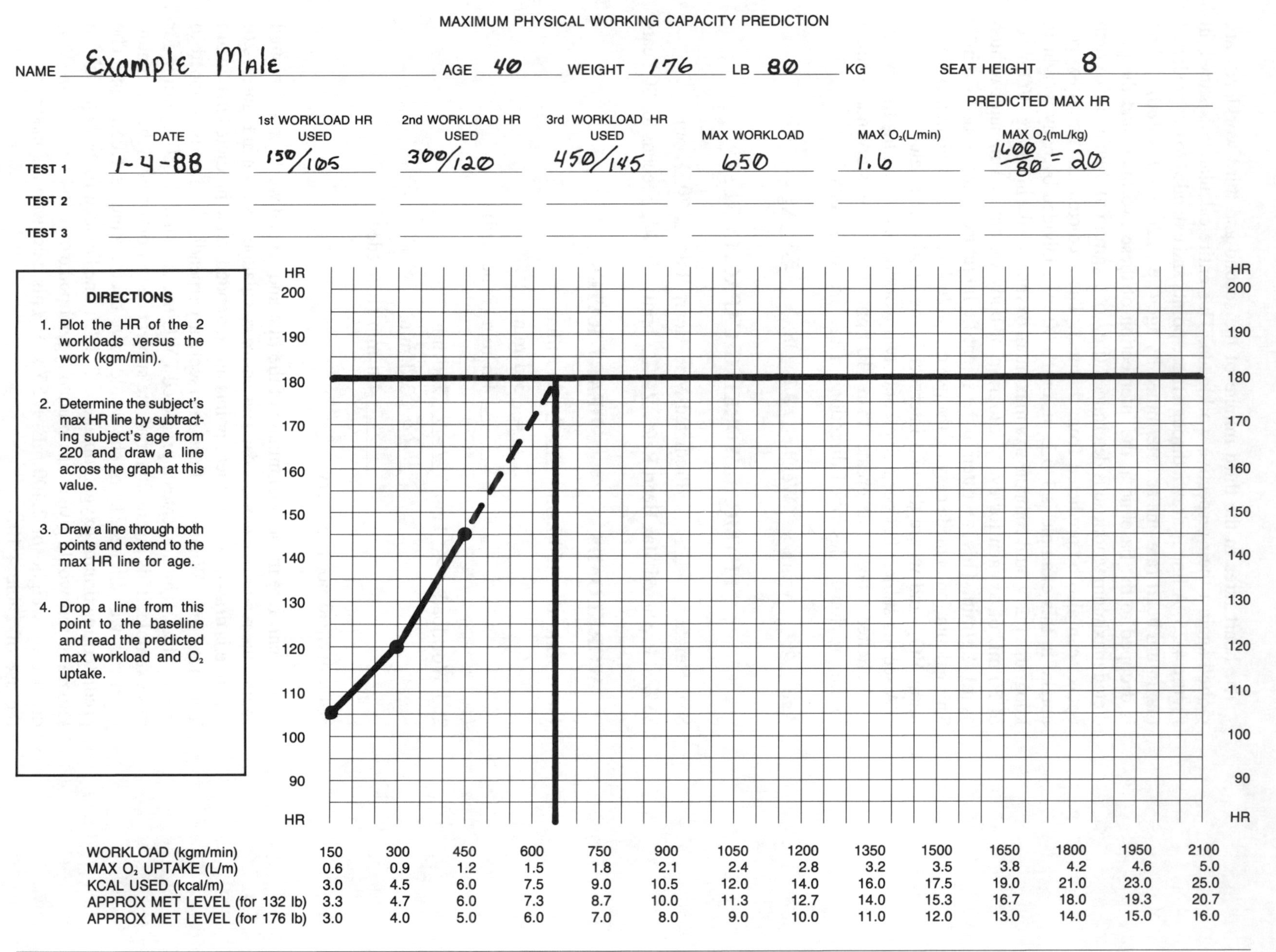

MAXIMUM PHYSICAL WORKING CAPACITY PREDICTION

NAME Example Male AGE 40 WEIGHT 176 LB 80 KG SEAT HEIGHT 8

PREDICTED MAX HR ______

	DATE	1st WORKLOAD HR USED	2nd WORKLOAD HR USED	3rd WORKLOAD HR USED	MAX WORKLOAD	MAX O_2(L/min)	MAX O_2(mL/kg)
TEST 1	1-4-88	150/105	300/120	450/145	650	1.6	1600/80 = 20
TEST 2							
TEST 3							

DIRECTIONS

1. Plot the HR of the 2 workloads versus the work (kgm/min).
2. Determine the subject's max HR line by subtracting subject's age from 220 and draw a line across the graph at this value.
3. Draw a line through both points and extend to the max HR line for age.
4. Drop a line from this point to the baseline and read the predicted max workload and O_2 uptake.

WORKLOAD (kgm/min)	150	300	450	600	750	900	1050	1200	1350	1500	1650	1800	1950	2100
MAX O_2 UPTAKE (L/m)	0.6	0.9	1.2	1.5	1.8	2.1	2.4	2.8	3.2	3.5	3.8	4.2	4.6	5.0
KCAL USED (kcal/m)	3.0	4.5	6.0	7.5	9.0	10.5	12.0	14.0	16.0	17.5	19.0	21.0	23.0	25.0
APPROX MET LEVEL (for 132 lb)	3.3	4.7	6.0	7.3	8.7	10.0	11.3	12.7	14.0	15.3	16.7	18.0	19.3	20.7
APPROX MET LEVEL (for 176 lb)	3.0	4.0	5.0	6.0	7.0	8.0	9.0	10.0	11.0	12.0	13.0	14.0	15.0	16.0

Figure 4-25. Sample graph plotted for three workloads.

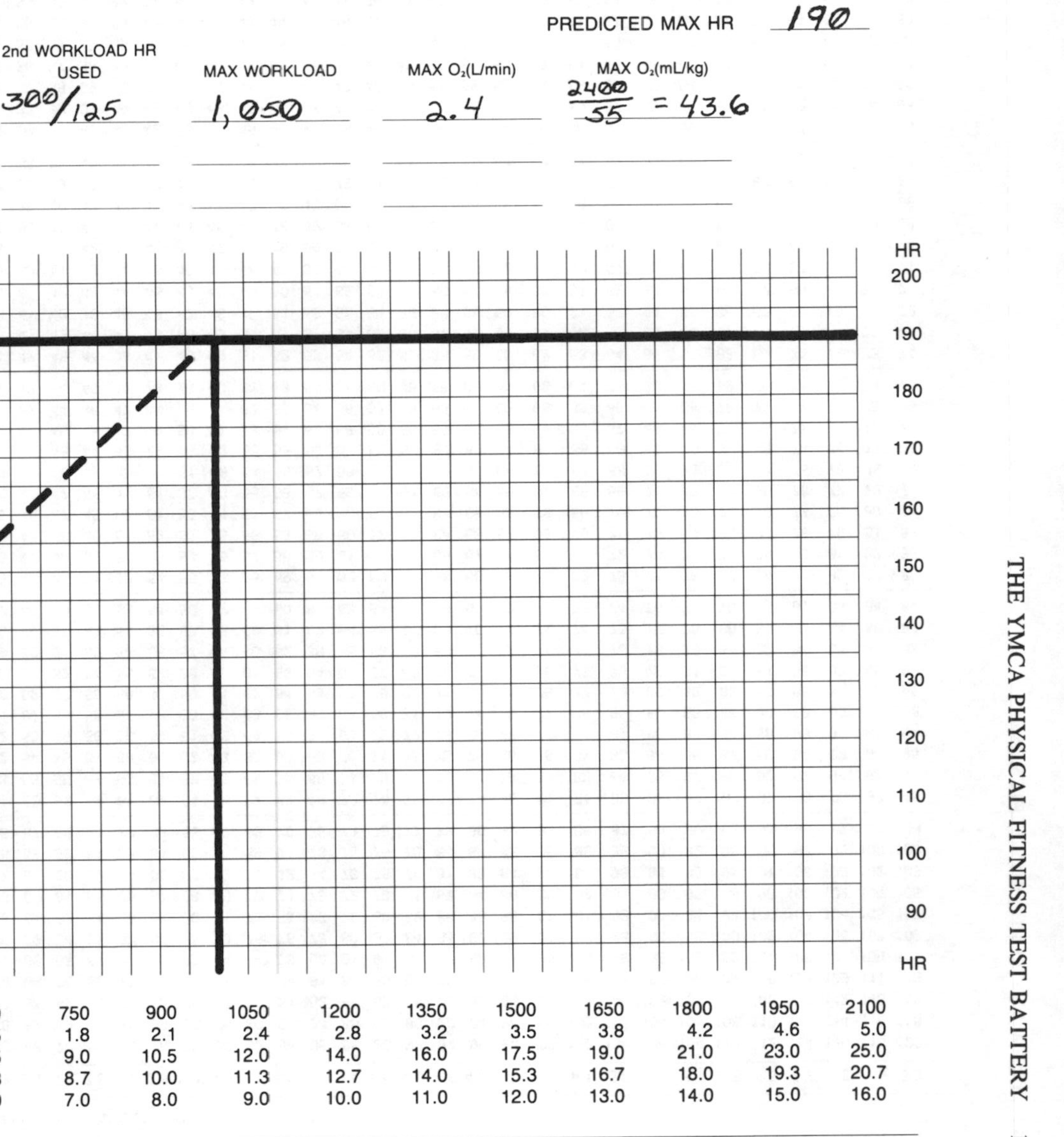

MAXIMUM PHYSICAL WORKING CAPACITY PREDICTION

NAME Example Female AGE 30 WEIGHT 121 LB 55 KG SEAT HEIGHT 6

PREDICTED MAX HR 190

	DATE	1st WORKLOAD HR USED	2nd WORKLOAD HR USED	MAX WORKLOAD	MAX O_2(L/min)	MAX O_2(mL/kg)
TEST 1	1-4-88	150/112	300/125	1,050	2.4	2400/55 = 43.6
TEST 2						
TEST 3						

DIRECTIONS

1. Plot the HR of the 2 workloads versus the work (kgm/min).
2. Determine the subject's max HR line by subtracting subject's age from 220 and draw a line across the graph at this value.
3. Draw a line through both points and extend to the max HR line for age.
4. Drop a line from this point to the baseline and read the predicted max workload and O_2 uptake.

WORKLOAD (kgm/min)	150	300	450	600	750	900	1050	1200	1350	1500	1650	1800	1950	2100
MAX O_2 UPTAKE (L/m)	0.6	0.9	1.2	1.5	1.8	2.1	2.4	2.8	3.2	3.5	3.8	4.2	4.6	5.0
KCAL USED (kcal/m)	3.0	4.5	6.0	7.5	9.0	10.5	12.0	14.0	16.0	17.5	19.0	21.0	23.0	25.0
APPROX MET LEVEL (for 132 lb)	3.3	4.7	6.0	7.3	8.7	10.0	11.3	12.7	14.0	15.3	16.7	18.0	19.3	20.7
APPROX MET LEVEL (for 176 lb)	3.0	4.0	5.0	6.0	7.0	8.0	9.0	10.0	11.0	12.0	13.0	14.0	15.0	16.0

Figure 4-26. Sample graph plotted for two workloads.

Table 4-10 Maximum Oxygen Uptake Conversion Chart (L/kg/min to mL/kg/min)

Body Weight		Maximum oxygen uptake (L/kg/min)																																											
lb	kg	1.5	1.6	1.7	1.8	1.9	2.0	2.1	2.2	2.3	2.4	2.5	2.6	2.7	2.8	2.9	3.0	3.1	3.2	3.3	3.4	3.5	3.6	3.7	3.8	3.9	4.0	4.1	4.2	4.3	4.4	4.5	4.6	4.7	4.8	4.9	5.0	5.1	5.2	5.3	5.4	5.5	5.6	5.7	5.8	5.9	6.0
110	50	30	32	34	36	38	40	42	44	46	48	50	52	54	56	58	60	62	64	66	68	70	72	74	76	78	80	82	84	86	88	90	92	94	96	98	100	102	104	106	108	110	112	114	116	118	120
112	51	29	31	33	35	37	39	41	43	45	47	49	51	53	55	57	59	61	63	65	67	69	71	73	75	76	78	80	82	84	86	88	90	92	94	96	98	100	102	104	106	108	110	112	114	116	118
115	52	29	31	33	35	37	38	40	42	44	46	48	50	52	54	56	58	60	62	63	65	67	69	71	73	75	77	79	81	83	85	87	88	90	92	94	96	98	100	102	104	106	108	110	112	113	115
117	53	28	30	32	34	36	38	40	42	43	45	47	49	51	53	55	57	58	60	62	64	66	68	70	72	74	75	77	79	81	83	85	87	89	91	92	94	96	98	100	102	104	106	108	109	111	113
119	54	28	30	31	33	35	37	39	41	43	44	46	48	50	52	54	56	57	59	61	63	65	67	69	70	72	74	76	78	80	81	83	85	87	89	91	93	94	96	98	100	102	104	106	107	109	111
121	55	27	29	31	33	35	36	38	40	42	44	45	47	49	51	53	55	56	58	60	62	64	65	.67	69	71	73	75	76	78	80	82	84	85	87	89	91	93	95	96	98	100	102	104	105	107	109
123	56	27	29	30	32	34	36	38	39	41	43	45	46	48	50	52	54	55	57	59	61	63	64	66	68	70	71	73	75	77	79	80	82	84	86	88	89	91	93	95	96	98	100	102	104	105	107
126	57	26	28	30	32	33	35	37	39	41	42	44	46	47	49	51	53	54	56	58	60	61	63	65	67	68	70	72	74	75	77	79	81	82	84	86	88	89	91	93	95	96	98	100	102	104	105
128	58	26	28	29	31	33	34	36	38	40	41	43	45	47	48	50	52	53	55	57	59	60	62	64	65	67	69	71	72	74	76	78	79	81	83	84	85	88	90	91	93	95	97	98	100	102	103
130	59	25	27	29	31	32	34	36	37	39	41	42	44	46	47	49	51	53	54	56	58	59	61	63	64	65	68	69	71	73	75	76	78	80	81	83	85	86	88	90	92	93	95	97	98	100	102
132	60	25	27	28	30	32	33	35	37	38	40	42	43	45	47	48	50	52	53	55	57	58	60	62	63	65	67	68	70	72	73	75	77	78	80	82	83	85	87	88	90	92	93	95	97	98	100
134	61	25	26	28	30	31	33	34	36	38	39	41	43	44	46	48	49	51	52	54	56	57	59	61	62	64	66	67	69	70	72	74	75	77	79	80	82	84	85	87	89	90	92	93	95	97	98
137	62	24	26	27	29	31	32	34	35	37	39	40	42	44	45	47	48	50	52	53	55	56	58	60	61	63	65	66	68	69	71	73	74	76	77	79	81	82	84	85	87	89	90	92	94	95	97
139	63	24	25	27	29	30	32	33	35	37	38	40	41	43	44	46	48	49	51	52	54	56	57	59	60	62	63	65	67	68	70	71	73	75	76	78	79	81	83	84	86	87	89	90	92	94	95
141	64	23	25	27	28	30	31	33	34	36	38	39	41	42	44	45	47	48	50	52	53	55	56	58	59	61	63	64	66	67	69	70	72	73	75	77	78	80	81	83	84	86	88	89	91	92	94
143	65	23	25	26	28	29	31	32	34	35	37	38	40	42	43	45	46	48	49	51	52	54	55	57	58	60	62	63	65	66	68	69	71	72	74	75	77	78	80	82	83	85	86	88	89	91	92
146	66	23	24	26	27	29	30	32	33	35	36	38	39	41	42	44	45	47	48	50	52	53	55	56	58	59	61	62	64	65	67	68	70	71	73	74	76	77	79	80	82	83	85	86	88	89	91
148	67	22	24	25	27	28	30	31	33	34	36	37	39	40	42	43	45	46	48	49	51	52	54	55	57	58	60	61	63	64	66	67	69	70	72	73	75	76	78	79	81	82	84	85	87	88	90
150	68	22	24	25	26	28	29	31	32	34	35	37	38	40	41	43	44	46	47	49	50	51	53	54	56	57	59	60	62	63	65	66	68	69	71	72	74	75	76	78	79	81	82	84	85	87	88
152	69	22	23	25	26	28	29	30	32	33	35	36	38	39	41	42	43	45	46	48	49	51	52	54	55	57	58	59	61	62	64	65	67	68	70	71	72	74	75	77	78	80	81	83	84	86	87
154	70	21	23	24	26	27	29	30	31	33	34	36	37	39	40	41	43	44	46	47	49	50	51	53	54	56	57	59	60	61	63	64	66	67	69	70	71	73	74	76	77	79	80	81	83	84	86
157	71	21	23	24	25	27	28	30	31	32	34	35	37	38	39	41	42	44	45	46	48	49	51	52	54	55	56	58	59	61	62	63	65	66	68	69	70	72	73	75	76	77	79	80	82	83	85
159	72	21	22	24	25	26	28	29	31	32	33	35	36	38	39	40	42	43	44	46	47	49	50	51	53	54	56	57	58	60	61	63	64	65	67	68	69	71	72	74	75	76	78	79	81	82	83
161	73	21	22	23	25	26	27	29	30	32	33	34	36	37	38	40	41	42	44	45	47	48	49	51	52	53	55	56	58	59	60	62	63	64	66	67	68	70	71	73	74	75	77	78	79	81	82
163	74	20	22	23	24	26	27	28	30	31	32	34	35	36	38	39	41	42	43	45	46	47	49	50	51	53	54	55	57	58	59	61	62	64	65	65	68	69	70	72	73	74	76	77	78	80	81
165	75	20	21	23	24	25	27	28	29	31	32	33	35	36	37	39	40	41	43	44	45	47	48	49	51	52	53	55	56	57	59	60	61	63	64	65	67	68	69	71	72	73	75	76	77	79	80
168	76	20	21	22	24	25	26	28	29	30	32	33	34	36	37	38	39	41	42	43	45	46	47	49	50	51	53	54	55	57	58	59	61	62	63	64	66	67	68	70	71	72	74	75	76	78	79
170	77	19	21	22	23	25	26	27	29	30	31	32	34	35	36	38	39	40	42	43	44	45	47	48	49	51	52	53	55	56	57	58	60	61	62	64	65	66	68	69	70	71	73	74	75	77	78
172	78	19	21	22	23	24	26	27	28	29	31	32	33	35	36	37	38	40	41	42	44	45	46	47	49	50	51	53	54	55	56	58	59	60	62	63	64	65	67	68	69	71	72	73	74	76	77
174	79	19	20	22	23	24	25	27	28	29	30	32	33	34	35	37	38	39	41	42	43	44	46	47	48	49	51	52	53	54	56	57	58	59	61	62	63	65	66	67	68	70	71	72	73	75	76
176	80	19	20	21	23	24	25	26	28	29	30	31	33	34	35	36	38	39	40	41	43	44	45	46	48	49	50	51	53	54	55	56	58	59	60	61	63	64	65	66	68	69	70	71	72	74	75
179	81	19	20	21	22	23	25	26	27	28	30	31	32	33	35	36	37	38	40	41	42	43	44	46	47	48	49	51	52	53	54	56	57	58	59	60	62	63	64	65	67	68	69	70	72	73	74
181	82	18	20	21	22	23	24	26	27	28	29	30	32	33	34	35	37	38	39	40	41	43	44	45	46	48	49	50	51	52	54	55	56	57	59	60	61	62	63	65	66	67	68	70	71	72	73
183	83	18	19	20	22	23	24	25	27	28	29	30	31	33	34	35	36	37	39	40	41	42	43	45	46	47	48	49	51	52	53	54	55	57	58	59	60	61	63	64	65	66	67	69	70	71	72
185	84	18	19	20	21	23	24	25	26	27	29	30	31	32	33	35	36	37	38	39	40	42	43	44	45	46	48	49	50	51	52	54	55	56	57	58	60	61	62	63	64	65	67	68	69	70	71
187	85	18	19	20	21	22	24	25	26	27	28	29	31	32	33	34	35	36	38	39	40	41	42	44	45	46	47	48	49	51	52	53	54	55	56	58	59	60	61	62	64	65	66	67	68	69	71
190	86	17	19	20	21	22	23	24	26	27	28	29	30	31	33	34	35	36	37	38	40	41	42	43	44	45	47	48	49	50	51	52	53	55	56	57	58	59	60	62	63	64	65	66	67	69	70
192	87	17	18	20	21	22	23	24	25	26	28	29	30	31	32	33	34	36	37	38	39	40	41	43	44	45	46	47	48	49	51	52	53	54	55	56	57	59	60	61	62	63	64	66	67	68	69
194	88	17	18	19	20	22	23	24	25	26	27	28	30	31	32	33	34	35	36	38	39	40	41	42	43	44	45	47	48	49	50	51	52	53	55	56	57	58	59	60	61	63	64	65	65	67	68
196	89	17	18	19	20	21	22	24	25	26	27	28	29	30	31	33	34	35	36	37	38	39	40	42	43	44	45	46	47	48	49	51	52	53	54	55	56	57	58	60	61	62	63	64	65	66	67
198	90	17	18	19	20	21	22	23	24	26	27	28	29	30	31	32	33	34	36	37	38	39	40	41	42	43	44	46	47	48	49	50	51	52	53	54	56	57	58	59	60	61	62	63	64	66	67
201	91	16	18	19	20	21	22	23	24	25	26	27	29	30	31	32	33	34	35	36	37	38	40	41	42	43	44	45	46	47	48	49	51	52	53	54	55	56	57	58	59	60	62	63	64	65	66
203	92	16	17	18	20	21	22	23	24	25	26	27	28	29	30	32	33	34	35	36	37	38	39	40	41	42	43	45	46	47	48	49	50	51	52	53	54	55	57	58	59	60	61	62	63	64	65
205	93	16	17	18	19	20	22	23	24	25	26	27	28	29	30	31	32	33	34	35	37	38	39	40	41	42	43	44	45	46	47	48	49	51	52	53	54	55	56	57	58	59	60	61	62	63	65
207	94	16	17	18	19	20	21	22	23	24	26	27	28	29	30	31	32	33	34	35	36	37	38	39	40	41	43	44	45	46	47	48	49	50	51	52	53	54	55	56	57	59	60	61	62	63	64
209	95	16	17	18	19	20	21	22	23	24	25	26	27	28	29	31	32	33	34	35	36	37	38	39	40	41	42	43	44	45	46	47	48	49	51	52	53	54	55	56	57	58	59	60	61	62	63
212	96	16	17	18	19	20	21	22	23	24	25	26	27	28	29	30	31	32	33	34	35	36	38	39	40	41	42	43	44	45	46	47	48	49	50	51	52	53	54	55	56	57	58	59	60	61	63
214	97	15	16	18	19	20	21	22	23	24	25	26	27	28	29	30	31	32	33	34	35	36	37	38	39	40	41	42	43	44	45	46	47	48	49	51	52	53	54	55	56	57	58	59	60	61	62
216	98	15	16	17	18	19	20	21	22	23	24	26	27	28	29	30	31	32	33	34	35	36	37	38	39	40	41	42	43	44	45	46	47	48	49	50	51	52	53	54	55	56	57	58	59	60	61
218	99	15	16	17	18	19	20	21	22	23	24	25	26	27	28	29	30	31	32	33	34	35	36	37	38	39	40	41	42	43	44	45	46	47	48	49	51	52	53	54	55	56	57	58	59	60	61
220	100	15	16	17	18	19	20	21	22	23	24	25	26	27	28	29	30	31	32	33	34	35	36	37	38	39	40	41	42	43	44	45	46	47	48	49	50	51	52	53	54	55	56	57	58	59	60

Note. From *Work Tests With the Bicycle Ergometer* (pp. 26-27) by P.-O. Åstrand, n.d., Varberg, Sweden: Monark. Copyright by Monark-Crescent AB. Reprinted by permission.

Test Interpretation

The YMCA bicycle ergometer test provides two measures that are useful in evaluating cardiovascular-respiratory function and working capacity: predicted maximum physical working capacity and predicted maximum oxygen uptake.

Both maximum physical working capacity and maximum oxygen uptake are discussed in chapter 3, which should be reviewed before interpreting test results to participants. Questions 42 through 51 are especially relevant.

Remember that these tests are estimates or predictions of maximal responses and have a greater chance of being in error than would be the case if the participants were exercised to their actual maximum. Interpretation must therefore be made carefully, and the possibility of poor or incorrect predictions must be understood.

Predicted Maximum Physical Working Capacity (PWC)

The predicted maximum PWC shows the workload at which the heart rate is expected to reach its maximum value. Assuming the test is done correctly, the greatest source of error is the possibility that the age-estimated maximum heart rate is not correct. Research has shown that the maximum heart rate has a wide range of values at any age. If the estimate is too high, maximum PWC will be overestimated; if it is too low, it will be underestimated. Accuracy can be improved if the true maximum heart rate is known. This is sometimes available if the participant has, for some reason, recently taken a stress ECG test. However, regardless of the possible errors, the norm tables are based on 220 minus age. If the norm tables are used, do not use the actual maximum heart rate even if it is known.

The greatest value in using the maximum PWC comes from comparing results before and after a participant enters an exercise program. Substantial improvement can be expected with participation in a YMCA exercise program conducted according to the established guidelines in chapter 5. Data can also be compared to norms presented at the end of this chapter.

Predicted Maximum Oxygen Uptake

The predicted maximum oxygen uptake is an extension of the PWC test. It is useful because there is so much interest in maximum oxygen uptake in current scientific and popular literature. As with the maximum PWC, improvement is expected with conditioning, and the results can be compared to available norms.

Assuming that the test is done correctly, the predicted maximum oxygen uptake is subject to the same source of errors as is the predicted maximum PWC, that is, the accuracy of the age-estimated maximum heart rate. There is also a second source of error. The oxygen uptake is calculated from the estimated maximum work rate. The assumption is that everyone expends the same amount of energy and uses the same amount of oxygen at a given work rate (energy expenditure is computed from the volume of oxygen used). The test will underestimate the true maximum for an individual who is very inefficient (expending a disproportionately large amount of energy to perform a given task) and will overestimate the true maximum oxygen uptake for an individual who is very efficient. Participants who are unfamiliar with bicycle exercise will tend to be less efficient than will those who bicycle regularly.

General Observations and Interpretation

As noted previously, both the maximum PWC and oxygen uptake can be compared to norms or used to demonstrate training effects; however, both are age dependent.

Use of the energy expenditure data in Appendix C is also important in interpreting results. By determining the MET and kilocalorie values from the chart, it is possible to anticipate an individual's response to exercise. According to the energy expenditure table in Appendix C, the first example subject's maximum working capacity, which is slightly greater than 8 Kcal per minute as estimated by the test, would be the equivalent of cycling at approximately 9.4 mph, but less than chopping wood fast, running 11.5-minute miles, or engaging in vigorous activity while skin diving. Examples of activities that require an expenditure of approximately 8 Kcal/min would be playing tennis or skiing in soft snow. If verticals are dropped at other heart rates, similar comparisons can be made.

No matter how the test results are used, the validity of the interpretation and the usefulness to the participant depend on obtaining high-quality data. The test must be given as described. The bicycle ergometer must be well maintained, which means regular calibration and proper maintenance. The environment must be well controlled, free from both physical and emotional stress. If there is any doubt about the results, test again to be sure.

The 3-Minute Step Test

Many YMCAs that are involved in corporate health enhancement programs or with other large groups have a need for mass testing of participants. Because of equipment needs, the bicycle is unsuited for this task. The 3-minute step test can be used very successfully in mass-testing situations. This is an excellent cardiorespiratory test not only for mass testing but also as a self-test or as an addition to a test battery. Minimal equipment is required, and participants can learn to administer it to themselves by counting the carotid or radial pulse; however, when done as a part of the test battery, it should be done as described here.

Equipment

1. A 12-in.-high, sturdy bench
2. A metronome set at 96 bpm (Four clicks of the metronome equal one step—up, up, down, down at 24 steps per minute. See the section in this chapter on metronomes.)
3. A timer for the 3 minutes and a timer for the recovery (these may be the same)
4. A stethoscope to count recovery heart rate
5. Testing forms to record data

Procedure

Demonstrate the stepping. Face the bench and, in time with the metronome, step one foot up on the bench (first beat), step up with the second foot (second beat), step down with the first foot (third beat), and step down with the other foot (fourth beat). The sequence is alternating feet. It does not matter which foot leads or if the lead foot changes during the test (see Fig. 4-27). Do not allow the participant to practice, as it will affect the heart rate.

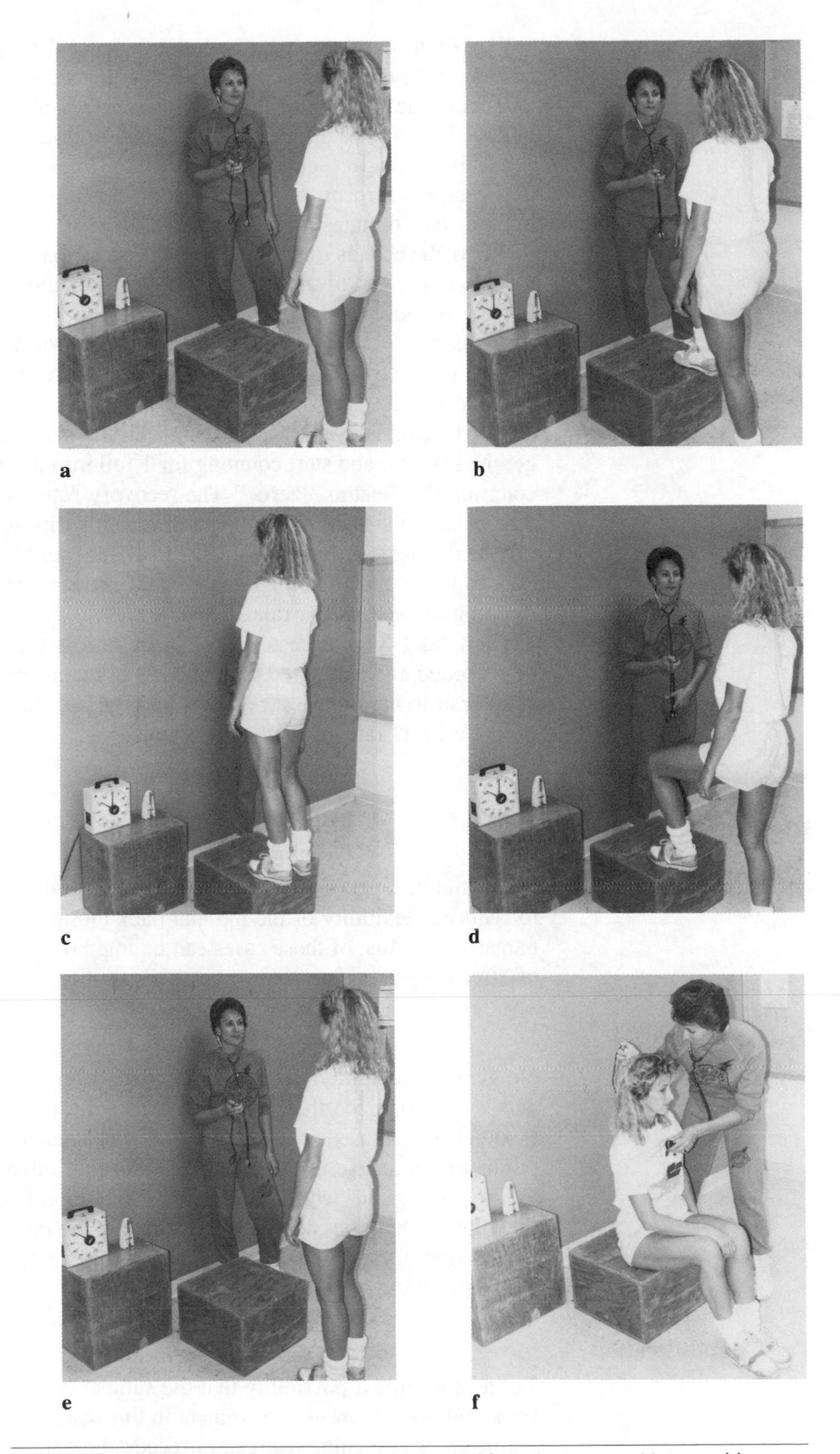

Figure 4-27. Three-minute step test. (a) Starting position; (b) step up; (c) up position; (d) step down; (e) down position; (f) heart-rate count.

Explain to the participant both the test and the importance of sitting down quickly at the end of 3 minutes and remaining still for 1 minute so that the tester can count the heart rate. Position the participant facing the bench and allow him or her to pick up the beat of the metronome by marking time in place. When the participant starts stepping, start the timer. Check the rhythm and correct if necessary. Inform the participant of the time as it passes by saying "One minute, two minutes," and so on.

When 20 seconds remain, remind the participant that he or she is to sit down quickly at the end of the stepping and wait for the tester to take the heart rate. Put the stethoscope in your ears and prepare the recovery timer. On the last step it is helpful to say "Last step—up, up, down, and sit."It might be helpful to turn the metronome off during the last 15 seconds stepping and count the cadence for the participant until the last step.

When the participant sits down, immediately place the stethoscope on the chest, get the rhythm, and start counting for 1 full minute. Begin the count on a beat, counting that beat as "zero." The recovery rate count must be started *within 5 seconds* or the heart rate will be significantly different. (Note: Pay close attention to the heart's rhythm, which can change suddenly during recovery. It is easy to lose count.) The 1-minute count reflects the heart's rate at the end of stepping as well as the rate of recovery.

The total 1-minute postexercise heart rate is the score for the test and can be recorded and compared to the norms in the scoring sheets at the end of this chapter or to previous test results if appropriate. Score the total 1-minute postexercise heart rate in beats per minute.

Flexibility Measurement

Many middle-aged people have low-back pain and disability. Often this is related to reduced flexibility of the hip and back along with reduced elasticity of the hamstrings. Most of these cases can be improved by a well-designed program of stretching exercises that increase flexibility.

Trunk Flexion

No general flexibility test exists that is representative of total body flexibility, and it is recognized that flexibility is specific to the joint in question. Trunk flexion has been used for the past 40 years as a general test of flexibility. Cureton published an article in 1941 on flexibility that introduced the Trunk Forward Flexion Test, and Scott and French (1959) modified the trunk flexion test in the 1950s. There has been a long history in the development and modification of this kind of flexibility test, the most recent being developed by Johnson and Nelson (1979).

Test Administration

There is a limited possibility that the subject could pull a muscle or strain the back with too vigorous a movement in this test. It is recommended that a short warm-up of stretching exercises precede the actual measurement and that the test be performed slowly and cautiously.

Equipment

1. A yardstick or tape measure to measure the distance reached, with a line drawn or taped on the floor at right angles to the 15-in. mark and the zero mark toward the participant
2. Tape to keep the measuring instrument in place on the floor and to mark a line
3. Testing forms to record data

Inexpensive, easily stored equipment can be built to facilitate convenient administration of this test (see Fig. 4-28). In addition, a commercially available trunk-flexion instrument can be successfully used (Fig. 4-29a, b).

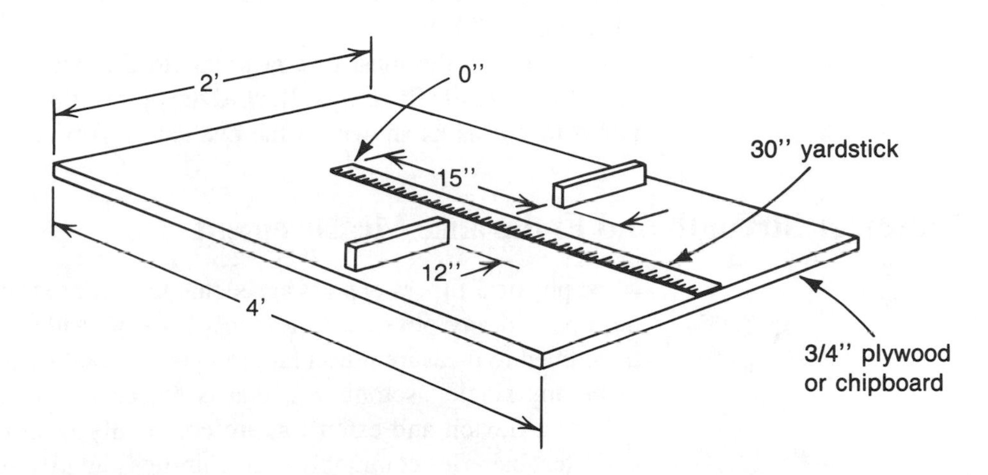

Figure 4-28. Hand-made flexibility board.

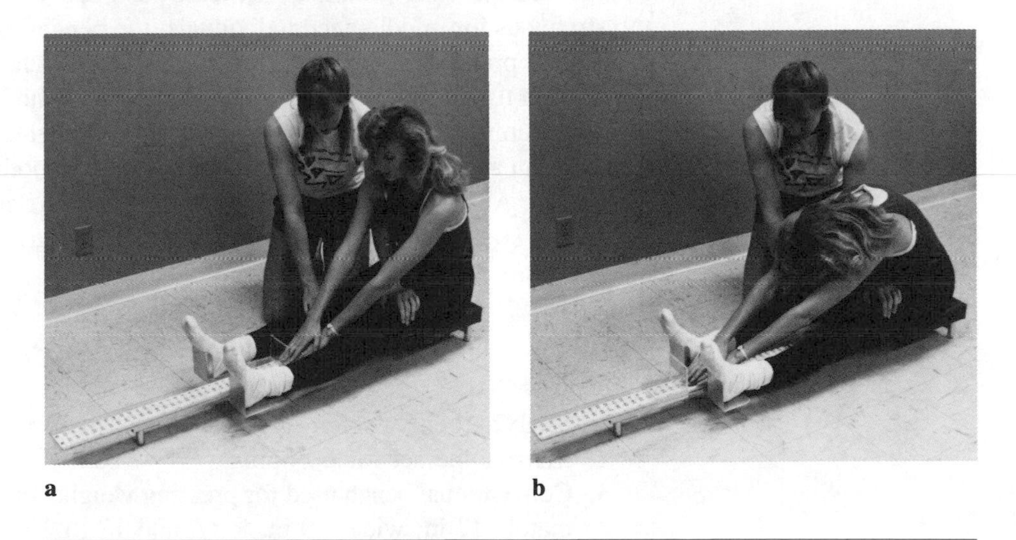

a b

Figure 4-29. Flexibility test. (a) Starting position; (b) stretching.

Procedure

In addition to warming-up prior to this test, participants also should refrain from fast, jerky movements that may increase the possibility of an injury.

Place a yardstick on the floor and put tape across it at right angles to the 15-in. mark. Have the participant sit with the yardstick between the legs with the 0 mark toward the body and the legs extended and abducted about 12 in. to the taped line on the floor. Shoes should be removed, and the heels of the feet should nearly touch the edge of the taped line and be about 10 to 12 in. apart (see Fig. 4-29a).

Have the participant slowly reach forward with both hands as far as possible on the yardstick, holding this position momentarily. To get the best stretch, the participant should exhale and drop the head between the arms when reaching. Be sure that the participant keeps the hands parallel and does not stretch or lead with one hand. Fingertips should be in contact with the yardstick. Insure that the participant's knees are kept straight by holding the knees down. (See Fig. 4-29b.)

The score is the most distant point (to the nearest 1/4 in.) reached on the yardstick with the fingertips. Record the best of three trials. Scores can be compared to norms as shown on the evaluation forms at the end of this chapter.

Muscular Strength and Endurance Measurement

Most physical fitness experts agree that muscular strength and endurance must be a part of any physical fitness test battery. Although many tests have been developed to measure muscular strength and endurance, there does not appear to be any single, isotonic test that is representative of total strength.

Elbow flexion and extension are commonly used to evaluate strength, and early test batteries commonly used chin-ups and push-ups as strength tests. The YMCA test battery uses elbow extension and spine and hip flexion to measure strength and muscular endurance. Because push-ups (elbow extension) are usually too strenuous for middle-aged individuals, the bench-press test was substituted. The bench press is elbow extension with a much lighter resistance than push-ups, which use body weight. The weights used in the bench press were determined by university and field testing to be the weights that normally could be lifted for an average of 15 repetitions, thus testing both muscular strength and endurance. Abdominal strength and its concomitant flat abdomen are desirable for adults, so timed sit-ups (spine and hip flexion) are used to test the strength and endurance of the abdominal muscles.

Bench Press Test

Equipment

1. 35-lb barbell (women); 80 lb barbell (men)
2. Metronome set for 60 bpm
3. Conventional bench used for pressing weights or a similar bench approximately 12 in. wide, 50 in. long, and 17 to 20 in. high (A lower bench should be built for shorter individuals.)
4. Testing forms to record data

Procedure

Have the participant lie on the bench in a supine (face up) position, with the knees bent and the feet on the floor. Hand the barbell to the participant, who has elbows flexed and palms up (down position). The participant should grip the bar with hands shoulder-width apart (see Fig. 4-30a). Have the participant then press the barbell upward to extend the elbows fully (see Fig. 4-30b). After each extension the participant should return the barbell to the original down position. The rhythm is kept by the metronome, with each click representing a movement up or down (60 bpm). Encourage the participants to breathe regularly and to not strain during the test to avoid the Valsalva maneuver.

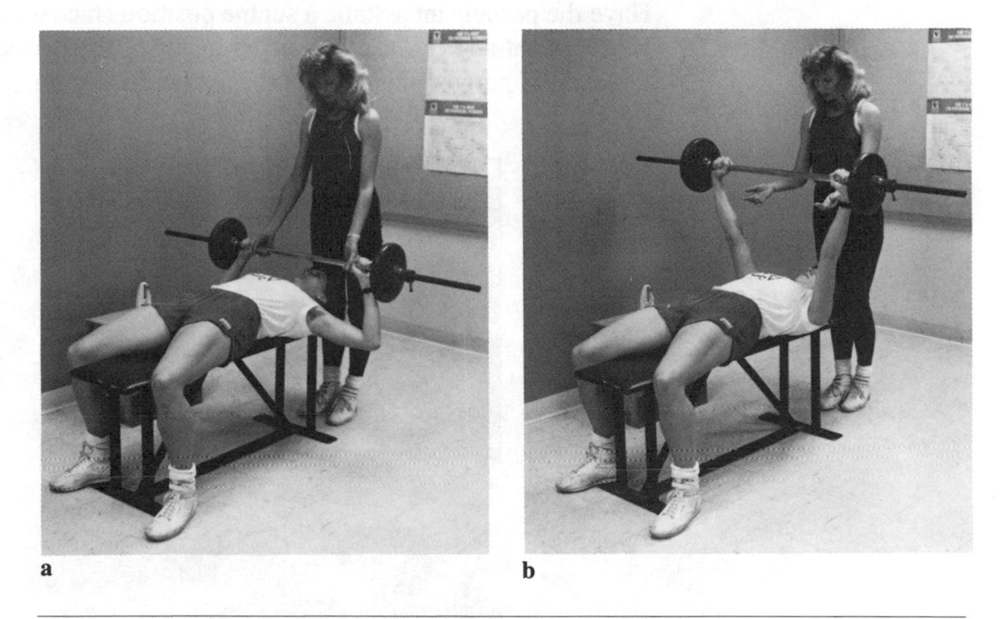

a b

Figure 4-30. Bench press test. (a) Starting position; (b) extension.

Scoring

Score the number of successful repetitions. The test is terminated when (a) a participant is unable to reach full extension of the elbows or (b) a participant breaks cadence and cannot keep up with the rhythm of the metronome.

For safety, at least one spotter should be present during the test. If a single spotter is physically unable to catch the weight, two spotters should be present, one at each end of the barbell.

1-Minute Timed Sit-Ups

As previously mentioned, muscular endurance is difficult to test due to the number of different muscles and muscle groups involved. Another problem is the subjective end point of most muscular endurance tests, which is somewhat dependent on motivation. Controlling the technique of execution used during testing is another difficulty. For these reasons the 1-minute timed sit-ups test was selected: It is fairly representative of general muscular endurance; it measures one of the most important muscle groups of the middle-aged individual; it is fairly standardized with respect to technique; and its 1-minute time period reduces the influence of motivation.

The use of full sit-ups as an exercise is controversial, and it is not being suggested that full sit-ups be used as an exercise in class. Half sit-ups, or crunches, exercise the abdominals better and do not put a strain on the lower back. However, to test abdominal strength and endurance, reliability can be obtained only if the test is done as explained, with the feet held and the body raised to a full sit-up position.

Equipment

1. Stopwatch or clock with a sweep second hand to time the sit-ups
2. A mat
3. Testing forms to record data

Procedure

Have the participant assume a supine position (face up) on the floor, with knees bent at right angles (heels about 18 in. from the buttocks) and fingers next to the ears. A partner should hold the ankles firmly for support (see Fig. 4-31a).

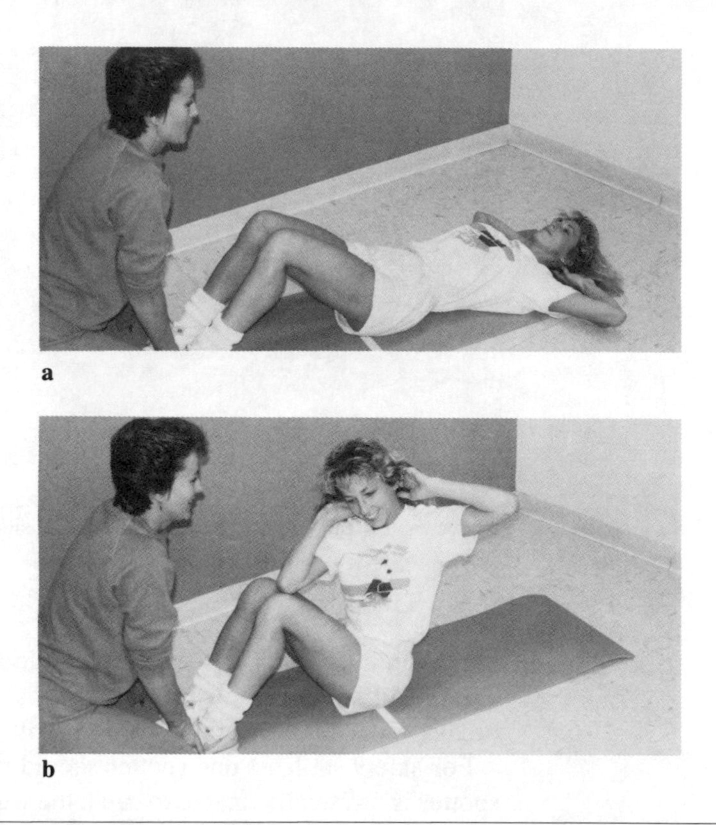

Figure 4-31. Sit-up test. (a) Down position; (b) up position.

At a "go" signal from the timer, have the participant then perform as many correct sit-ups as possible within a 1-minute period. The elbows should alternately touch the opposite knee as the participant comes into the up position (see Fig. 4-31b). The partner should maintain the count. After each up movement the participant should return to the supine position before going up again; shoulders must be returned to touch the mat, but the head need not touch. Score the number of repetitions in 1 minute. (Caution: The participant should breathe easily during the exercise so as not to invoke the Valsalva maneuver.)

Y's Way to Physical Fitness

Physical Fitness Evaluation Profile

Norms—Men 18-25

Name ______________________ Dates: T1 ________ T2 ________ T3 ________

Rating	% ranking	Resting HR	% fat	3-min step test	PWC max (kgm)	$\dot{V}O_2$max (mL/kg)	Flexibility	Bench press	Sit-ups
Excellent	100	49	4	70	2350	80	26	45	60
	95	52	6	72	2275	71	22	42	54
	90	55	7	78	2065	63	20	38	50
Good	85	57	8	82	1905	59	20	34	48
	80	60	9	85	1795	55	19	32	46
	75	61	10	88	1705	53	18	30	45
Above average	70	63	11	91	1630	51	18	28	42
	65	64	12	94	1570	49	17	26	41
	60	65	13	97	1515	47	17	25	40
Average	55	67	14	101	1455	46	16	22	38
	50	68	15	102	1400	45	16	22	37
	45	69	16	104	1350	43	15	21	36
Below average	40	71	18	107	1305	41	14	20	34
	35	72	19	110	1260	39	14	17	33
	30	73	20	114	1195	38	13	16	32
Poor	25	76	22	118	1135	35	12	13	30
	20	79	24	121	1090	33	12	12	28
	15	81	26	126	1050	31	10	9	26
Very poor	10	84	28	131	975	29	9	8	24
	5	89	30	137	885	26	7	2	17
	0	95	37	164	850	20	2	0	12

Actual Scores									
	T1	____	____	____	____	____	____	____	____
	T2	____	____	____	____	____	____	____	____
	T3	____	____	____	____	____	____	____	____

	T1	T2	T3
Actual Weight	________	________	________
Target Weight	________	________	________
Blood Pressure	____/____	____/____	____/____

Your actual weight should be within 10% of your target weight. If your blood pressure exceeds 150/90 it is considered high. Your YMCA Medical Advisory Committee should have guidelines for when blood pressure is too high to continue fitness testing.

Y's Way to Physical Fitness

Physical Fitness Evaluation Profile

Norms—Men 26-35

Name ______________________ Dates: T1 ________ T2 ________ T3 ________

Rating	% ranking	Resting HR	% fat	3-min step test	PWC max (kgm)	$\dot{V}O_2$max (mL/kg)	Flexibility	Bench press	Sit-ups
Excellent	100 95 90	49 52 54	8 10 12	73 76 79	2300 2180 1950	70 64 58	25 22 20	43 40 34	55 50 46
Good	85 80 75	57 60 61	13 14 15	83 85 88	1820 1740 1665	54 52 50	19 18 18	30 29 26	45 42 41
Above average	70 65 60	62 64 65	16 17 18	91 94 97	1600 1545 1485	47 46 44	17 17 16	25 24 22	38 37 36
Average	55 50 45	66 68 70	19 20 21	101 103 106	1430 1375 1325	42 41 40	16 15 15	21 20 18	34 33 32
Below average	40 35 30	72 73 74	22 23 24	109 113 116	1270 1225 1180	39 38 35	14 13 12	17 14 13	30 30 29
Poor	25 20 15	77 78 81	25 26 28	119 122 126	1135 1080 1020	34 33 31	12 11 10	12 10 9	28 25 24
Very poor	10 5 0	84 88 94	30 32 37	130 140 164	960 840 780	28 26 20	9 7 2	5 2 0	21 12 6

Actual Scores									
	T1	____	____	____	____	____	____	____	____
	T2	____	____	____	____	____	____	____	____
	T3	____	____	____	____	____	____	____	____

	T1	T2	T3
Actual Weight	________	________	________
Target Weight	________	________	________
Blood Pressure	/	/	/

Your actual weight should be within 10% of your target weight. If your blood pressure exceeds 150/90 it is considered high. Your YMCA Medical Advisory Committee should have guidelines for when blood pressure is too high to continue fitness testing.

Y's Way to Physical Fitness

Physical Fitness Evaluation Profile

Norms—Men 36-45

Name ______________________ Dates: T1 ________ T2 ________ T3 ________

Rating	% ranking	Resting HR	% fat	3-min step test	PWC max (kgm)	$\dot{V}O_2max$ (mL/kg)	Flexibility	Bench press	Sit-ups
	100	50	10	72	2250	77	24	40	50
Excellent	95	53	12	74	2055	60	21	34	46
	90	56	14	81	1815	53	19	30	42
	85	60	16	86	1725	49	19	28	40
Good	80	61	17	90	1640	46	17	25	37
	75	62	18	94	1565	44	17	24	36
	70	64	19	98	1500	42	17	22	34
Above average	65	65	20	100	1440	41	15	21	32
	60	66	21	102	1375	40	15	20	30
	55	68	22	105	1325	38	15	18	29
Average	50	69	23	108	1280	37	14	17	29
	45	70	24	111	1235	35	13	16	28
	40	73	25	113	1190	34	13	14	26
Below average	35	74	26	116	1140	33	11	13	25
	30	76	26	118	1090	32	11	12	24
	25	77	27	120	1045	30	11	10	22
Poor	20	80	28	124	995	28	9	9	20
	15	82	29	128	945	27	9	8	18
	10	86	30	132	860	25	7	5	16
Very poor	5	90	32	142	745	21	5	2	9
	0	96	38	168	700	19	1	0	4

Actual Scores T1 ____ ____ ____ ____ ____ ____ ____ ____

T2 ____ ____ ____ ____ ____ ____ ____ ____

T3 ____ ____ ____ ____ ____ ____ ____ ____

	T1	T2	T3
Actual Weight	________	________	________
Target Weight	________	________	________
Blood Pressure	___/___	___/___	___/___

Your actual weight should be within 10% of your target weight. If your blood pressure exceeds 150/90 it is considered high. Your YMCA Medical Advisory Committee should have guidelines for when blood pressure is too high to continue fitness testing.

Y's Way to Physical Fitness

Physical Fitness Evaluation Profile

Norms—Men 46-55

Name ______________________ Dates: T1 ________ T2 ________ T3 ________

Rating	% ranking	Resting HR	% fat	3-min step test	PWC max (kgm)	$\dot{V}O_2max$ (mL/kg)	Flexibility	Bench press	Sit-ups
Excellent	100	50	12	78	2150	60	23	35	50
	95	53	14	81	1940	54	20	28	41
	90	57	16	84	1645	47	19	24	36
Good	85	59	18	89	1520	43	17	22	33
	80	60	19	93	1450	42	17	21	30
	75	63	20	96	1385	40	16	20	29
Above average	70	64	21	99	1335	38	15	17	28
	65	65	22	101	1285	36	15	16	26
	60	67	23	103	1240	35	14	14	25
Average	55	68	24	109	1205	35	13	13	24
	50	69	24	113	1165	34	12	12	22
	45	71	25	115	1130	32	12	10	22
Below average	40	73	26	118	1090	31	11	10	21
	35	75	27	120	1055	30	10	9	20
	30	76	28	121	1020	29	10	8	18
Poor	25	79	29	124	950	28	9	6	17
	20	80	30	126	935	27	8	5	16
	15	83	31	130	885	26	7	4	13
Very poor	10	85	32	135	830	23	6	2	12
	5	91	34	145	750	22	4	1	8
	0	97	38	158	700	18	1	0	4
Actual Scores	T1	____	____	____	____	____	____	____	____
	T2	____	____	____	____	____	____	____	____
	T3	____	____	____	____	____	____	____	____

	T1	T2	T3
Actual Weight	________	________	________
Target Weight	________	________	________
Blood Pressure	____/____	____/____	____/____

Your actual weight should be within 10% of your target weight. If your blood pressure exceeds 150/90 it is considered high. Your YMCA Medical Advisory Committee should have guidelines for when blood pressure is too high to continue fitness testing.

Y's Way to Physical Fitness

Physical Fitness Evaluation Profile

Norms—Men 56-65

Name ______________________ Dates: T1 ________ T2 ________ T3 ________

Rating	% ranking	Resting HR	% fat	3-min step test	PWC max (kgm)	$\dot{V}O_2max$ (mL/kg)	Flexibility	Bench press	Sit-ups
Excellent	100	51	15	72	2100	58	21	32	42
	95	52	17	74	1665	49	19	24	37
	90	56	18	82	1485	43	17	22	32
Good	85	59	19	89	1400	39	17	20	29
	80	60	20	93	1315	38	15	18	28
	75	61	21	97	1240	37	15	14	26
Above average	70	64	22	98	1195	35	13	14	24
	65	65	23	100	1150	34	13	12	22
	60	67	24	101	1100	33	13	10	21
Average	55	68	24	105	1055	31	11	10	20
	50	69	25	109	1005	31	11	8	18
	45	71	26	111	965	30	11	8	17
Below average	40	72	26	113	925	29	9	6	16
	35	73	27	116	890	27	9	6	14
	30	75	28	118	860	26	9	4	13
Poor	25	76	29	122	830	25	7	4	12
	20	79	30	125	795	23	7	2	10
	15	81	31	128	740	22	5	2	9
Very poor	10	84	32	131	680	21	5	0	8
	5	88	34	136	597	18	3	0	4
	0	94	38	150	590	16	1	0	2

Actual Scores									
	T1	____	____	____	____	____	____	____	____
	T2	____	____	____	____	____	____	____	____
	T3	____	____	____	____	____	____	____	____

	T1	T2	T3
Actual Weight	________	________	________
Target Weight	________	________	________
Blood Pressure	____/____	____/____	____/____

Your actual weight should be within 10% of your target weight. If your blood pressure exceeds 150/90 it is considered high. Your YMCA Medical Advisory Committee should have guidelines for when blood pressure is too high to continue fitness testing.

Y's Way to Physical Fitness

Physical Fitness Evaluation Profile

Norms—Men Over 65

Name ______________________ Dates: T1 __________ T2 __________ T3 __________

Rating	% ranking	Resting HR	% fat	3-min step test	PWC max (kgm)	$\dot{V}O_2$max (mL/kg)	Flexibility	Bench press	Sit-ups
Excellent	100	50	15	72	1940	50	20	30	40
	95	53	17	74	1405	42	18	20	33
	90	55	18	86	1235	38	17	18	29
Good	85	58	19	89	1175	36	15	14	26
	80	59	20	92	1110	34	14	12	25
	75	61	21	95	1045	33	13	10	22
Above average	70	62	22	97	1015	32	13	10	21
	65	63	22	100	990	30	12	10	21
	60	65	23	102	945	29	11	8	20
Average	55	66	24	104	900	28	11	8	18
	50	69	24	109	870	26	10	6	17
	45	69	25	113	840	25	9	6	16
Below average	40	70	25	114	805	25	9	4	14
	35	71	26	116	765	24	8	4	13
	30	73	27	119	725	22	8	4	12
Poor	25	75	28	122	695	21	7	2	10
	20	77	29	126	665	21	6	2	9
	15	79	30	128	610	20	5	2	8
Very poor	10	83	31	133	555	18	4	0	6
	5	89	33	140	510	17	3	0	4
	0	98	38	152	490	15	0	0	2

Actual Scores									
	T1	____	____	____	____	____	____	____	____
	T2	____	____	____	____	____	____	____	____
	T3	____	____	____	____	____	____	____	____

	T1	T2	T3
Actual Weight	________	________	________
Target Weight	________	________	________
Blood Pressure	___/___	___/___	___/___

Your actual weight should be within 10% of your target weight. If your blood pressure exceeds 150/90 it is considered high. Your YMCA Medical Advisory Committee should have guidelines for when blood pressure is too high to continue fitness testing.

Y's Way to Physical Fitness

Physical Fitness Evaluation Profile

Norms—Women 18-25

Name ______________________ Dates: T1 ________ T2 ________ T3 ________

Rating	% ranking	Resting HR	% fat	3-min step test	PWC max (kgm)	$\dot{V}O_2$max (mL/kg)	Flexibility	Bench press	Sit-ups
Excellent	100 95 90	54 56 60	13 15 17	72 79 83	1830 1640 1440	71 67 58	27 25 24	50 42 36	55 48 44
Good	85 80 75	61 64 65	18 19 20	88 93 97	1320 1235 1175	54 50 48	23 22 21	32 29 28	41 38 37
Above average	70 65 60	66 68 69	21 22 23	100 103 106	1120 1075 1030	46 43 42	21 20 20	25 24 22	36 34 33
Average	55 50 45	70 72 73	24 25 25	110 112 116	990 950 915	41 40 39	19 19 18	21 20 18	32 30 29
Below average	40 35 30	74 76 78	26 27 28	118 122 124	880 845 810	37 35 34	18 17 17	16 14 13	28 26 25
Poor	25 20 15	80 82 84	29 30 31	128 133 137	775 740 705	32 31 29	16 15 14	12 9 8	24 22 20
Very poor	10 5 0	86 90 100	33 37 43	142 149 155	640 555 500	26 22 18	13 12 8	5 2 1	17 10 4

Actual Scores T1 ____ ____ ____ ____ ____ ____ ____ ____

T2 ____ ____ ____ ____ ____ ____ ____ ____

T3 ____ ____ ____ ____ ____ ____ ____ ____

	T1	T2	T3
Actual Weight	______	______	______
Target Weight	______	______	______
Blood Pressure	___/___	___/___	___/___

Your actual weight should be within 10% of your target weight. If your blood pressure exceeds 150/90 it is considered high. Your YMCA Medical Advisory Committee should have guidelines for when blood pressure is too high to continue fitness testing.

Y's Way to Physical Fitness

Physical Fitness Evaluation Profile

Norms—Women 26-35

Name ______________________ Dates: T1 ________ T2 ________ T3 ________

Rating	% ranking	Resting HR	% fat	3-min step test	PWC max (kgm)	$\dot{V}O_2$max (mL/kg)	Flexibility	Bench press	Sit-ups
Excellent	100	54	13	72	1800	69	26	48	54
	95	55	15	80	1440	59	24	40	42
	90	59	18	86	1330	54	23	33	40
Good	85	60	19	91	1245	51	22	29	37
	80	63	20	93	1180	48	21	26	34
	75	64	21	97	1115	46	20	25	33
Above average	70	66	22	103	1065	43	20	22	32
	65	67	23	106	1020	42	19	21	30
	60	68	23	110	985	40	19	20	29
Average	55	69	24	112	955	38	18	18	28
	50	70	25	116	925	37	18	17	26
	45	71	26	118	885	35	18	16	25
Below average	40	72	27	121	840	34	17	14	24
	35	74	29	124	805	33	16	13	23
	30	76	30	127	765	31	16	12	21
Poor	25	78	31	129	730	30	15	9	20
	20	80	33	131	695	28	14	8	18
	15	82	35	135	655	26	14	5	16
Very poor	10	84	36	141	600	25	13	2	12
	5	88	39	148	530	22	11	1	2
	0	94	49	154	490	20	8	0	1
Actual Scores	T1	____	____	____	____	____	____	____	____
	T2	____	____	____	____	____	____	____	____
	T3	____	____	____	____	____	____	____	____

	T1	T2	T3
Actual Weight	________	________	________
Target Weight	________	________	________
Blood Pressure	____/____	____/____	____/____

Your actual weight should be within 10% of your target weight. If your blood pressure exceeds 150/90 it is considered high. Your YMCA Medical Advisory Committee should have guidelines for when blood pressure is too high to continue fitness testing.

Y's Way to Physical Fitness

Physical Fitness Evaluation Profile

Norms—Women 36-45

Name ____________________ Dates: T1 ________ T2 ________ T3 ________

Rating	% ranking	Resting HR	% fat	3-min step test	PWC max (kgm)	$\dot{V}O_2max$ (mL/kg)	Flexibility	Bench press	Sit-ups
Excellent	100 95 90	54 56 59	15 17 19	74 80 87	1780 1360 1215	66 53 46	25 23 22	46 32 28	50 38 34
Good	85 80 75	62 63 64	20 21 23	93 97 101	1135 1085 1035	44 41 39	21 20 19	25 22 21	30 29 27
Above average	70 65 60	66 68 69	24 25 26	104 106 109	980 925 880	37 36 34	19 18 17	20 18 17	26 25 24
Average	55 50 45	70 71 72	27 28 29	111 114 117	835 800 765	33 32 31	17 16 16	14 13 12	22 21 20
Below average	40 35 30	74 76 78	30 31 32	120 122 127	745 720 695	30 29 28	15 15 14	11 10 9	18 17 16
Poor	25 20 15	79 80 82	33 35 36	130 135 138	670 625 575	26 25 23	13 12 11	8 6 4	14 12 10
Very poor	10 5 0	84 88 92	39 41 48	143 146 152	530 490 470	21 19 18	10 9 6	2 1 0	6 2 1

Actual Scores									
	T1	____	____	____	____	____	____	____	____
	T2	____	____	____	____	____	____	____	____
	T3	____	____	____	____	____	____	____	____

	T1	T2	T3
Actual Weight	________	________	________
Target Weight	________	________	________
Blood Pressure	____/____	____/____	____/____

Your actual weight should be within 10% of your target weight. If your blood pressure exceeds 150/90 it is considered high. Your YMCA Medical Advisory Committee should have guidelines for when blood pressure is too high to continue fitness testing.

Y's Way to Physical Fitness

Physical Fitness Evaluation Profile

Norms—Women 46-55

Name ______________________ Dates: T1 ________ T2 ________ T3 ________

Rating	% ranking	Resting HR	% fat	3-min step test	PWC max (kgm)	$\dot{V}O_2max$ (mL/kg)	Flexibility	Bench press	Sit-ups
Excellent	100	54	18	76	1700	64	24	42	42
	95	56	19	88	1245	48	22	30	30
	90	60	22	93	1130	42	21	26	28
Good	85	61	23	96	1045	39	20	22	25
	80	64	24	100	980	36	19	21	24
	75	65	25	102	930	35	18	20	22
Above average	70	66	26	106	885	33	18	17	21
	65	68	27	111	850	32	17	14	20
	60	69	28	113	815	31	17	13	18
Average	55	70	29	117	790	30	16	12	17
	50	72	30	118	760	29	16	11	16
	45	73	31	120	730	28	15	10	14
Below average	40	74	32	121	700	27	15	9	13
	35	76	33	124	670	26	14	8	12
	30	77	34	126	640	25	14	6	10
Poor	25	78	36	127	610	24	13	5	9
	20	81	37	131	585	23	12	4	8
	15	84	38	133	545	21	11	2	6
Very poor	10	85	40	138	495	19	10	1	4
	5	90	42	147	430	18	8	0	1
	0	96	49	152	400	16	4	0	0

Actual Scores T1 ____ ____ ____ ____ ____ ____ ____ ____

T2 ____ ____ ____ ____ ____ ____ ____ ____

T3 ____ ____ ____ ____ ____ ____ ____ ____

	T1	T2	T3
Actual Weight	________	________	________
Target Weight	________	________	________
Blood Pressure	____/____	____/____	____/____

Your actual weight should be within 10% of your target weight. If your blood pressure exceeds 150/90 it is considered high. Your YMCA Medical Advisory Committee should have guidelines for when blood pressure is too high to continue fitness testing.

Y's Way to Physical Fitness

Physical Fitness Evaluation Profile

Norms—Women 56-65

Name ______________________ Dates: T1 ________ T2 ________ T3 ________

Rating	% ranking	Resting HR	% fat	3-min step test	PWC max (kgm)	$\dot{V}O_2$max (mL/kg)	Flexibility	Bench press	Sit-ups
Excellent	100	54	18	74	1650	57	23	34	38
	95	56	20	83	1165	43	21	30	29
	90	59	23	92	1015	38	20	22	25
Good	85	61	24	97	970	36	19	20	21
	80	63	25	99	895	34	18	18	20
	75	64	26	103	840	32	18	16	18
Above average	70	67	28	106	790	31	17	15	17
	65	68	29	109	750	30	17	14	14
	60	69	30	111	720	28	16	12	13
Average	55	71	31	113	690	27	15	10	12
	50	72	32	116	660	26	15	9	11
	45	73	33	117	635	25	15	8	10
Below average	40	75	34	119	605	24	14	7	9
	35	76	35	123	575	23	13	6	8
	30	77	36	127	550	22	13	4	7
Poor	25	79	36	129	530	21	12	3	6
	20	80	37	132	510	20	11	2	5
	15	81	38	136	475	19	10	1	4
Very poor	10	85	39	142	420	17	9	0	2
	5	89	42	148	355	15	7	0	1
	0	96	46	151	340	14	3	0	0

Actual Scores T1 ____ ____ ____ ____ ____ ____ ____ ____

T2 ____ ____ ____ ____ ____ ____ ____ ____

T3 ____ ____ ____ ____ ____ ____ ____ ____

	T1	T2	T3
Actual Weight	________	________	________
Target Weight	________	________	________
Blood Pressure	____/____	____/____	____/____

Your actual weight should be within 10% of your target weight. If your blood pressure exceeds 150/90 it is considered high. Your YMCA Medical Advisory Committee should have guidelines for when blood pressure is too high to continue fitness testing.

Y's Way to Physical Fitness

Physical Fitness Evaluation Profile

Norms—Women Over 65

Name ______________________ Dates: T1 ________ T2 ________ T3 ________

Rating	% ranking	Resting HR	% fat	3-min step test	PWC max (kgm)	$\dot{V}O_2$max (mL/kg)	Flexibility	Bench press	Sit-ups
Excellent	100	54	16	73	1190	51	22	26	36
	95	56	17	83	860	39	21	22	26
	90	59	18	86	820	33	20	18	24
Good	85	60	22	93	725	31	19	14	22
	80	62	23	97	665	30	18	13	20
	75	64	25	100	640	28	18	12	18
Above average	70	66	27	104	610	27	17	11	16
	65	67	28	108	585	26	17	10	15
	60	68	29	114	560	25	16	9	14
Average	55	70	30	117	540	24	15	8	13
	50	71	31	120	525	23	15	6	12
	45	72	32	121	510	22	14	5	11
Below average	40	73	33	123	495	22	13	4	10
	35	75	34	126	480	21	13	3	8
	30	76	35	127	470	20	12	2	6
Poor	25	79	36	129	460	18	11	2	4
	20	80	37	132	425	17	10	1	3
	15	84	38	134	395	17	9	0	2
Very poor	10	88	39	135	370	16	8	0	1
	5	91	40	149	340	15	6	0	0
	0	96	44	151	320	14	2	0	0

Actual Scores									
	T1	____	____	____	____	____	____	____	____
	T2	____	____	____	____	____	____	____	____
	T3	____	____	____	____	____	____	____	____

	T1	T2	T3
Actual Weight	________	________	________
Target Weight	________	________	________
Blood Pressure	___/___	___/___	___/___

Your actual weight should be within 10% of your target weight. If your blood pressure exceeds 150/90 it is considered high. Your YMCA Medical Advisory Committee should have guidelines for when blood pressure is too high to continue fitness testing.

Y's Way to Physical Fitness

Body Composition Profile

Norms—Men 18-25

Name ______________________ Dates: T1 ________ T2 ________ T3 ________

Rating	% ranking	% fat	Chest (mm)	Abdomen (mm)	Ilium (mm)	Axilla (mm)	Tricep (mm)	Back (mm)	Thigh (mm)
Very lean	100	4	3	5	4	3	3	4	5
	95	6	3	7	5	4	4	5	6
	90	7	4	9	8	5	5	7	7
Lean	85	8	5	11	9	6	6	8	8
	80	9	6	12	10	7	7	9	9
	75	10	7	13	12	8	8	9	10
Leaner than average	70	11	8	16	13	9	8	10	11
	65	12	8	17	14	10	9	11	12
	60	13	9	19	16	11	10	12	13
Average	55	14	10	21	17	12	10	12	14
	50	15	11	23	18	14	11	13	14
	45	16	12	24	21	16	12	13	15
Fatter than average	40	18	13	27	22	17	12	14	16
	35	19	15	28	24	18	13	15	17
	30	20	16	31	26	20	14	16	18
Fat	25	22	17	33	29	21	15	17	19
	20	24	20	37	33	22	16	18	20
	15	26	23	41	36	25	18	21	22
Over fat	10	28	25	45	38	29	20	24	26
	5	30	32	51	44	36	24	30	30
	0	37	42	66	58	46	30	46	38

Actual Scores									
	T1	____	____	____	____	____	____	____	____
	T2	____	____	____	____	____	____	____	____
	T3	____	____	____	____	____	____	____	____

Y's Way to Physical Fitness

Body Composition Profile

Norms—Men 26-35

Name ______________________ Dates: T1 ________ T2 ________ T3 ________

Rating	% ranking	% fat	Chest (mm)	Abdomen (mm)	Ilium (mm)	Axilla (mm)	Tricep (mm)	Back (mm)	Thigh (mm)
Very lean	100	8	4	8	6	4	4	6	6
	95	10	5	10	8	6	5	7	7
	90	12	6	15	11	9	6	8	9
Lean	85	13	7	17	12	10	7	8	10
	80	14	8	19	14	11	8	9	11
	75	15	9	21	16	12	8	11	13
Leaner than average	70	16	10	22	18	13	9	12	14
	65	17	11	23	19	14	10	13	15
	60	18	12	25	20	16	11	14	16
Average	55	19	13	26	23	17	12	15	17
	50	20	14	28	24	18	13	16	17
	45	21	15	30	26	19	14	16	18
Fatter than average	40	22	16	31	28	20	14	17	19
	35	23	17	33	30	21	15	18	20
	30	24	19	35	31	22	16	19	21
Fat	25	25	21	37	34	25	17	20	23
	20	26	23	41	35	26	18	21	25
	15	28	25	42	39	29	20	24	27
Over fat	10	30	27	46	43	32	20	28	30
	5	32	29	50	48	34	24	33	32
	0	37	42	68	55	46	34	46	48

Actual Scores

T1 ____ ____ ____ ____ ____ ____ ____ ____

T2 ____ ____ ____ ____ ____ ____ ____ ____

T3 ____ ____ ____ ____ ____ ____ ____ ____

Y's Way to Physical Fitness

Body Composition Profile

Norms—Men 36-45

Name ______________________ Dates: T1 ________ T2 ________ T3 ________

Rating	% ranking	% fat	Chest (mm)	Abdomen (mm)	Ilium (mm)	Axilla (mm)	Tricep (mm)	Back (mm)	Thigh (mm)
Very lean	100	10	4	8	6	5	4	6	6
	95	12	5	11	8	8	5	7	7
	90	14	8	17	12	10	7	9	9
Lean	85	16	9	19	15	12	8	10	10
	80	17	11	22	16	13	9	11	12
	75	18	12	25	17	14	10	12	13
Leaner than average	70	19	13	26	20	16	11	14	14
	65	20	15	27	21	17	11	15	15
	60	21	16	29	23	18	12	16	16
Average	55	22	17	30	24	19	13	17	17
	50	23	18	31	25	20	13	18	17
	45	24	19	33	27	21	14	19	18
Fatter than average	40	25	20	34	28	22	14	20	19
	35	26	21	37	31	23	15	22	20
	30	26	23	38	32	24	16	23	21
Fat	25	27	24	39	33	25	17	24	22
	20	28	25	42	36	26	18	26	23
	15	29	28	45	39	29	19	28	25
Over fat	10	30	31	47	41	32	21	32	29
	5	32	35	51	45	34	25	38	33
	0	38	46	68	50	42	32	44	44

Actual Scores

T1 ____ ____ ____ ____ ____ ____ ____ ____

T2 ____ ____ ____ ____ ____ ____ ____ ____

T3 ____ ____ ____ ____ ____ ____ ____ ____

Y's Way to Physical Fitness

Body Composition Profile

Norms—Men 46-55

Name ______________________ Dates: T1 ________ T2 ________ T3 ________

Rating	% ranking	% fat	Chest (mm)	Abdomen (mm)	Ilium (mm)	Axilla (mm)	Tricep (mm)	Back (mm)	Thigh (mm)
Very lean	100	12	5	10	8	7	4	6	6
	95	14	7	13	9	9	6	9	7
	90	16	8	17	12	10	7	10	9
Lean	85	18	11	20	14	11	8	12	10
	80	19	12	22	16	13	9	13	11
	75	20	13	24	18	14	10	14	12
Leaner than average	70	21	15	26	20	15	10	16	13
	65	22	16	28	21	17	11	17	14
	60	23	17	29	22	18	12	18	15
Average	55	24	18	30	23	19	12	19	16
	50	24	19	32	25	21	13	20	17
	45	25	20	33	26	22	14	21	18
Fatter than average	40	26	21	34	28	23	14	22	19
	35	27	23	37	29	25	15	24	21
	30	28	24	38	30	26	16	25	22
Fat	25	29	27	41	33	27	17	26	23
	20	30	28	44	34	29	18	28	25
	15	31	29	46	37	31	19	30	26
Over fat	10	32	33	49	41	34	20	33	30
	5	34	37	53	44	38	24	37	33
	0	38	46	64	56	48	32	46	44

Actual Scores

T1 ____ ____ ____ ____ ____ ____ ____ ____

T2 ____ ____ ____ ____ ____ ____ ____ ____

T3 ____ ____ ____ ____ ____ ____ ____ ____

Y's Way to Physical Fitness

Body Composition Profile

Norms—Men 56-65

Name ______________________ Dates: T1 ________ T2 ________ T3 ________

Rating	% ranking	% fat	Chest (mm)	Abdomen (mm)	Ilium (mm)	Axilla (mm)	Tricep (mm)	Back (mm)	Thigh (mm)
Very lean	100	15	5	12	7	9	4	7	6
	95	17	7	16	9	11	6	9	7
	90	18	10	19	12	12	7	11	8
Lean	85	19	12	22	13	13	8	12	9
	80	20	14	23	14	14	9	13	10
	75	21	15	24	17	15	10	14	11
Leaner than average	70	22	16	26	18	16	10	15	13
	65	23	17	27	19	17	11	17	14
	60	24	18	28	20	18	12	18	15
Average	55	24	19	29	21	19	13	19	16
	50	25	19	30	22	20	14	20	17
	45	26	20	31	24	21	14	21	18
Fatter than average	40	26	22	32	25	22	14	22	19
	35	27	23	34	26	23	15	23	20
	30	28	24	36	28	25	16	24	21
Fat	25	29	27	38	29	26	17	25	22
	20	30	28	40	30	27	18	27	23
	15	31	31	43	33	29	20	29	25
Over fat	10	32	34	46	36	32	22	31	27
	5	34	38	51	41	37	26	35	33
	0	38	48	60	54	44	30	46	38

Actual Scores									
	T1	____	____	____	____	____	____	____	____
	T2	____	____	____	____	____	____	____	____
	T3	____	____	____	____	____	____	____	____

Y's Way to Physical Fitness

Body Composition Profile

Norms—Men Over 65

Name ______________________ Dates: T1 ________ T2 ________ T3 ________

Rating	% ranking	% fat	Chest (mm)	Abdomen (mm)	Ilium (mm)	Axilla (mm)	Tricep (mm)	Back (mm)	Thigh (mm)
Very lean	100	15	7	10	6	7	4	6	6
	95	17	9	13	8	9	5	9	7
	90	18	10	15	9	11	6	10	8
Lean	85	19	12	17	10	12	7	11	9
	80	20	13	18	12	13	8	12	10
	75	21	14	19	13	14	9	13	11
Leaner than average	70	22	15	21	14	15	10	14	12
	65	22	16	22	16	17	10	15	13
	60	23	17	23	17	18	11	16	14
Average	55	24	18	25	18	19	11	17	15
	50	24	19	26	19	20	12	18	15
	45	25	20	27	20	21	12	19	15
Fatter than average	40	25	21	29	21	21	13	20	16
	35	26	22	30	22	22	13	21	17
	30	27	24	31	24	23	14	22	17
Fat	25	28	25	33	25	25	15	23	18
	20	29	26	35	26	27	16	24	19
	15	30	26	38	28	29	17	25	21
Over fat	10	31	30	39	30	31	18	26	23
	5	33	33	47	36	35	19	32	27
	0	38	42	56	46	42	20	36	30

Actual Scores									
	T1	____	____	____	____	____	____	____	____
	T2	____	____	____	____	____	____	____	____
	T3	____	____	____	____	____	____	____	____

Y's Way to Physical Fitness

Body Composition Profile

Norms—Women 18-25

Name ______________________ Dates: T1 ________ T2 ________ T3 ________

Rating	% ranking	% fat	Chest (mm)	Abdomen (mm)	Ilium (mm)	Axilla (mm)	Tricep (mm)	Back (mm)	Thigh (mm)
Very lean	100 95 90	13 15 17	4 5 6	7 9 10	4 6 8	6 8 9	7 9 11	5 7 8	13 15 16
Lean	85 80 75	18 19 20	7 8 9	13 14 15	10 11 12	10 10 11	12 13 14	9 10 11	19 20 21
Leaner than average	70 65 60	21 22 23	10 11 12	16 17 18	13 14 16	12 12 13	15 16 17	11 12 12	22 23 24
Average	55 50 45	24 25 25	12 13 14	19 21 22	17 18 19	13 14 14	18 19 19	13 13 14	25 26 27
Fatter than average	40 35 30	26 27 28	15 16 17	23 25 26	20 21 22	15 16 16	20 21 22	15 16 17	28 30 31
Fat	25 20 15	29 30 31	18 20 21	27 30 31	25 26 28	17 18 20	23 25 26	18 19 21	32 35 38
Over fat	10 5 0	33 37 43	22 26 38	34 39 52	32 36 50	22 24 34	29 33 42	23 28 36	40 46 52

Actual Scores

T1 ____ ____ ____ ____ ____ ____ ____ ____

T2 ____ ____ ____ ____ ____ ____ ____ ____

T3 ____ ____ ____ ____ ____ ____ ____ ____

Y's Way to Physical Fitness

Body Composition Profile

Norms—Women 26-35

Name ______________________ Dates: T1 __________ T2 __________ T3 __________

Rating	% ranking	% fat	Chest (mm)	Abdomen (mm)	Ilium (mm)	Axilla (mm)	Tricep (mm)	Back (mm)	Thigh (mm)
Very lean	100	13	3	6	4	4	8	4	13
	95	15	3	8	5	6	10	6	15
	90	18	4	11	8	7	11	7	19
Lean	85	19	5	12	9	8	13	8	20
	80	20	6	15	11	9	14	9	21
	75	21	7	16	12	10	15	10	23
Leaner than average	70	22	8	17	13	10	16	11	24
	65	23	9	18	14	11	17	12	25
	60	23	10	19	15	11	18	13	27
Average	55	24	11	20	16	12	18	14	28
	50	25	12	21	17	12	19	15	29
	45	26	13	24	20	13	20	16	31
Fatter than average	40	27	14	25	21	14	21	16	32
	35	29	15	27	23	15	22	17	33
	30	30	17	28	25	16	23	18	35
Fat	25	31	19	31	27	17	25	19	36
	20	33	21	33	29	18	27	20	37
	15	35	23	35	32	24	29	22	40
Over fat	10	36	25	37	37	26	31	26	43
	5	39	35	44	43	30	34	30	47
	0	48	42	58	58	34	48	40	62

Actual Scores									
	T1	____	____	____	____	____	____	____	____
	T2	____	____	____	____	____	____	____	____
	T3	____	____	____	____	____	____	____	____

Y's Way to Physical Fitness

Body Composition Profile

Norms—Women 36-45

Name ______________________ Dates: T1 ________ T2 ________ T3 ________

Rating	% ranking	% fat	Chest (mm)	Abdomen (mm)	Ilium (mm)	Axilla (mm)	Tricep (mm)	Back (mm)	Thigh (mm)
Very lean	100	15	3	7	5	6	8	4	15
	95	17	3	9	7	8	10	6	17
	90	19	5	12	8	9	12	8	19
Lean	85	20	6	14	11	10	14	9	22
	80	21	7	16	12	11	15	10	23
	75	23	9	18	13	12	16	12	25
Leaner than average	70	24	11	20	15	13	17	13	26
	65	25	13	21	16	14	18	14	27
	60	26	14	22	17	14	19	15	29
Average	55	27	15	24	19	15	20	16	30
	50	28	16	25	20	16	21	17	31
	45	29	17	26	21	18	22	18	33
Fatter than average	40	30	18	29	23	20	23	19	34
	35	31	19	32	24	21	24	20	35
	30	32	20	33	27	22	26	22	38
Fat	25	33	21	34	28	23	27	24	39
	20	35	25	37	31	24	28	25	42
	15	36	27	40	33	28	31	28	46
Over fat	10	39	31	44	37	32	32	33	50
	5	41	35	49	41	34	38	36	55
	0	48	40	60	50	44	44	46	66

Actual Scores

T1 ____ ____ ____ ____ ____ ____ ____ ____

T2 ____ ____ ____ ____ ____ ____ ____ ____

T3 ____ ____ ____ ____ ____ ____ ____ ____

Y's Way to Physical Fitness

Body Composition Profile

Norms—Women 46-55

Name ______________________ Dates: T1 ________ T2 ________ T3 ________

Rating	% ranking	% fat	Chest (mm)	Abdomen (mm)	Ilium (mm)	Axilla (mm)	Tricep (mm)	Back (mm)	Thigh (mm)
Very lean	100 95 90	18 19 22	2 3 4	10 12 18	5 6 9	6 8 9	10 14 15	6 8 10	12 16 19
Lean	85 80 75	23 24 25	5 7 9	19 20 23	11 14 15	10 12 13	16 17 18	11 12 14	22 23 24
Leaner than average	70 65 60	26 27 28	11 12 13	24 26 28	17 18 19	14 15 16	19 20 21	15 16 17	27 28 30
Average	55 50 45	29 30 31	15 16 17	29 30 31	22 23 25	18 19 20	22 23 24	18 19 20	31 32 34
Fatter than average	40 35 30	32 33 34	19 20 21	32 35 38	26 27 29	21 22 23	25 27 28	22 23 24	35 38 40
Fat	25 20 15	36 37 38	24 25 28	39 42 46	30 33 37	24 28 29	30 31 34	26 28 31	43 46 50
Over fat	10 5 0	40 42 49	31 36 46	48 52 60	39 45 60	30 34 38	36 40 52	35 38 52	52 58 68

Actual Scores									
	T1	____	____	____	____	____	____	____	____
	T2	____	____	____	____	____	____	____	____
	T3	____	____	____	____	____	____	____	____

Y's Way to Physical Fitness

Body Composition Profile

Norms—Women 56-65

Name ______________________ Dates: T1 ________ T2 ________ T3 ________

Rating	% ranking	% fat	Chest (mm)	Abdomen (mm)	Ilium (mm)	Axilla (mm)	Tricep (mm)	Back (mm)	Thigh (mm)
Very lean	100 95 90	18 20 23	3 3 4	10 13 18	8 10 11	8 10 12	10 11 14	7 8 10	10 11 18
Lean	85 80 75	24 25 26	5 6 8	21 23 26	12 15 16	14 15 16	17 18 19	11 12 14	22 25 26
Leaner than average	70 65 60	28 29 30	9 12 14	29 30 31	17 20 21	18 19 20	21 22 23	15 16 17	28 29 30
Average	55 50 45	31 32 33	16 19 22	33 34 35	23 24 25	21 22 23	24 25 26	18 19 20	31 34 37
Fatter than average	40 35 30	34 35 36	23 24 25	37 38 41	27 28 29	24 25 26	27 28 29	21 22 23	38 39 41
Fat	25 20 15	36 37 38	27 28 31	42 43 46	31 33 36	27 30 31	30 31 34	24 26 28	42 43 46
Over fat	10 5 0	39 42 46	32 33 50	49 53 60	39 44 58	32 36 48	37 39 52	30 36 44	49 53 60

Actual Scores									
	T1	____	____	____	____	____	____	____	____
	T2	____	____	____	____	____	____	____	____
	T3	____	____	____	____	____	____	____	____

Y's Way to Physical Fitness

Body Composition Profile

Norms—Women Over 65

Name ______________________ Dates: T1 __________ T2 __________ T3 __________

Rating	% ranking	% fat	Chest (mm)	Abdomen (mm)	Ilium (mm)	Axilla (mm)	Tricep (mm)	Back (mm)	Thigh (mm)
Very lean	100	16	3	7	5	7	7	6	7
	95	17	3	9	6	9	8	8	9
	90	18	4	13	8	10	12	9	13
Lean	85	22	5	17	10	11	14	10	17
	80	23	6	21	12	12	15	11	20
	75	25	7	24	14	13	16	12	23
Leaner than average	70	27	10	25	16	13	17	13	24
	65	28	11	26	17	14	18	14	25
	60	29	12	28	19	15	19	15	29
Average	55	30	13	30	20	19	20	16	31
	50	31	14	32	21	20	22	17	32
	45	32	15	33	22	21	23	18	34
Fatter than average	40	33	17	36	24	22	24	18	35
	35	34	20	37	26	23	25	19	36
	30	35	21	35	28	25	26	20	37
Fat	25	36	22	41	29	27	27	21	38
	20	37	23	44	30	28	28	22	39
	15	38	26	46	33	29	30	23	44
Over fat	10	39	27	49	36	30	32	24	48
	5	40	33	53	41	31	35	30	55
	0	44	40	58	54	34	44	36	62

Actual Scores T1 ____ ____ ____ ____ ____ ____ ____ ____

T2 ____ ____ ____ ____ ____ ____ ____ ____

T3 ____ ____ ____ ____ ____ ____ ____ ____

Y's Way to Physical Fitness

SCORE SHEET—MEN

NAME ______________________ DATE __________

TIME __________

Age ________ years Weight ________ lb ________ kg Height ________ in.

Resting Blood Pressure ________/________ mm Hg Resting Heart Rate ________ bpm

1. SKINFOLDS

Chest ________ mm

Abdomen ________ mm

Ilium ________ mm

Axilla ________ mm

Scapula ________ mm

Tricep ________ mm

Thigh ________ mm

2. PERCENT FAT

Sum of 4		Sum of 3	
Abdomen	________	Abdomen	________
Ilium	________	Ilium	________
Tricep	________	Tricep	________
Thigh	________	**Sum**	________
Sum	________		
Percent fat	________ %	Percent fat	________ %

3. TARGET WEIGHT (16% fat) ________ lb

4. PHYSICAL WORK CAPACITY TEST

Seat Height ________ Predicted Max Heart Rate ________ bpm

85% of Predicted Max Heart Rate ________ bpm ________ Seconds for 30 Beats

WORKLOADS	HEART RATES
1st Workload 150 kgm	________ 2nd min
	________ 3rd min
	________ 4th min (if needed)
2nd Workload ________ kgm	________ 2nd min
	________ 3rd min
	________ 4th min (if needed)
3rd Workload ________ kgm	________ 2nd min
	________ 3rd min
	________ 4th min (if needed)

Transfer above results to the PWC graph and compute.

5. FLEXIBILITY

Trunk Flexion ________ in.

6. MUSCULAR STRENGTH & ENDURANCE

Bench Press (80 lb) ________ reps

1-Minute Timed Sit-Ups ________ reps

Transfer results to the Physical Fitness Evaluation Profile and the Body Composition Profile.

Y's Way to Physical Fitness

SCORE SHEET—WOMEN

NAME ______________________________ DATE __________

TIME __________

Age ________ years Weight ________ lb ________ kg Height ________ in.

Resting Blood Pressure ________/________ mm Hg Resting Heart Rate ________ bpm

---

1. SKINFOLDS

Chest ________ mm

Abdomen ________ mm

Ilium ________ mm

Axilla ________ mm

Scapula ________ mm

Tricep ________ mm

Thigh ________ mm

2. PERCENT FAT

Sum of 4		Sum of 3	
Abdomen	________	Abdomen	________
Ilium	________	Ilium	________
Tricep	________	Tricep	________
Thigh	________	**Sum**	________
Sum	________		
Percent fat	________ %	Percent fat	________ %

3. TARGET WEIGHT (23% fat) ________ lb

4. PHYSICAL WORK CAPACITY TEST

Seat Height ________ Predicted Max Heart Rate ________ bpm

85% of Predicted Max Heart Rate ________ bpm ________ Seconds for 30 Beats

WORKLOADS	HEART RATES
1st Workload 150 kgm	________ 2nd min
	________ 3rd min
	________ 4th min (if needed)
2nd Workload ________ kgm	________ 2nd min
	________ 3rd min
	________ 4th min (if needed)
3rd Workload ________ kgm	________ 2nd min
	________ 3rd min
	________ 4th min (if needed)

Transfer above results to the PWC graph and compute.

5. FLEXIBILITY

Trunk Flexion ________ in.

6. MUSCULAR STRENGTH & ENDURANCE

Bench Press (35 lb) ________ reps

1-Minute Timed Sit-Ups ________ reps

Transfer results to the Physical Fitness Evaluation Profile and the Body Composition Profile.

Exercise Principles and Guidelines

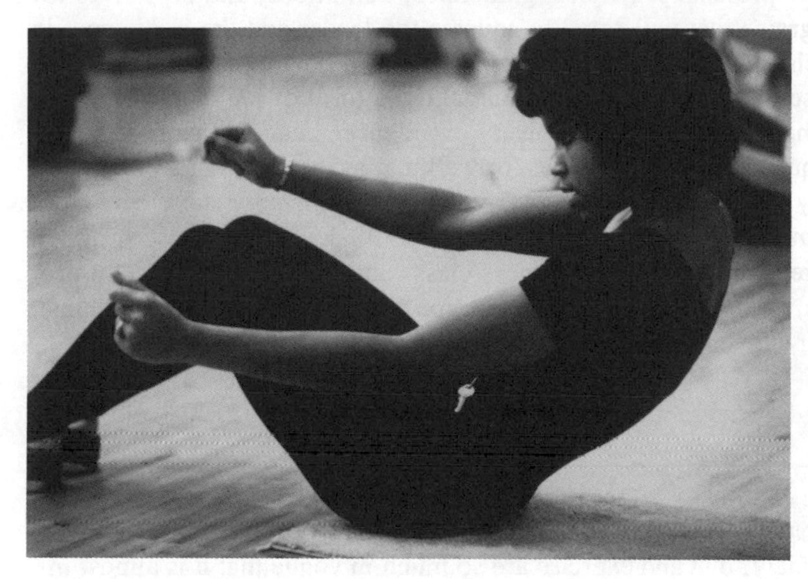

Chapter 5

The national YMCA physical fitness programs have many facets—planning, organization, testing and evaluation, and programming—all of which are important. Testing is important because it determines the fitness status of each individual, shows the fitness areas that need particular emphasis, and illustrates the dramatic changes and improvement that occur as a result of fitness program participation. Workshops and other training events emphasize the test battery and train potential leaders in the fine points of administering it. However, of all the various facets of the programs, the actual exercises that a Y member participates in are the core, the central focus, of the national programs.

The exercise program guidelines and principles presented in this chapter are suitable for any exercise program, although they are primarily geared to the unfit, middle-aged adult who has not recently participated in regular physical activity. A conservative approach to exercise is recommended when starting sedentary adults on exercise. Contraindications to exercise must be determined by medical evaluation, after which a slow progression will prevent many of the undesirable effects of sudden and too strenuous exercise.

Many principles discussed in this chapter are general, but they deal mostly with adult group programs conducted in a large area such as a gymnasium, requiring little or no equipment and no special skills from the participants. The purpose of this chapter is not to present an outline or list of exercises nor to offer a progression in actual number of repetitions. The exercises selected by the leader should be determined by the types of people in the class, the facilities, the available equipment, and the leader's previous experience. Ingenuity, variety, and enthusiasm are attributes that cannot be taught; they come through genuine interest, experience, and desire.

This chapter presents principles, guidelines, definitions, and objectives for exercise programs that will serve to educate the leader and the participant in how to exercise, what to expect from exercise, and how to exercise on one's own. Exercise in the YMCA setting can take the form of jogging, weightlifting, swimming, cycling, or any of many excellent recreational games such as tennis or racquetball. (Exercise plans for walking, swimming, outdoor cycling, and stationary cycling are available in *Health Enhancement for America's Work Force—Program Guide* [YMCA of the USA, 1987].) The exercise program discussed here is the more formal fitness-class routine. This is the type of program that can be used to help people become fit so that they can play tennis, ski, swim, or just enjoy life more.

PHYSICAL FITNESS

In today's society, diet and exercise are so much in vogue that it is almost impossible to attend any social, professional, or even family gathering without hearing people mention what new diet they are on, how many miles they run each day, or what health spa they have just joined; yet the American public is getting fatter each year. The health spa business and the diet industry are booming. It is estimated that 40% of Americans are overweight, which translates to 75 to 80 million people. It is also estimated that half of these people are trying to do something about their obesity, but the dropout rate for health spas is over 50%. There still are those who are not in systematic, progressive programs; and there still are health clubs that recommend passive devices such as rollers, vibrating belts, or saunas to achieve weight loss, muscle tone, and fitness.

In recent years, people's reasons for exercising have become fairly exotic. They exercise to lose weight, to reduce the incidence of coronary heart disease, to cure or prevent low-back pain, to lessen stress, to live longer, to retain youth, or to look more athletic. These are all desirable outcomes, and some are possible and others impossible to reach. The inability of fad diets and passive exercise to achieve and maintain participants' goals seems to suggest that the problem of fitness is not being attacked in the proper way. People expect instant results with little effort. Most people spend years getting out of shape (if indeed they ever were in shape) and expect to regain their youthful, fit figures in a few weeks. This lack of instant fitness causes many new fitness enthusiasts to stop exercising after a few weeks.

Dieters follow much the same pattern; the lack of substantial weight loss after a relatively short period of dieting discourages them, and they soon return to their former eating habits. Dozens of fad diets have met with little success because their claims are unrealistic and, in a few cases, potentially harmful. Without behavior change, which means changing one's basic eating habits permanently, lost weight is usually quickly regained when former eating habits are resumed.

It has probably taken years to become obese, and many dieters expect to attain their target weight after only a few weeks of dieting. We need to apply the basic principles of exercise and good nutrition to obtain desired results.

What Is Physical Fitness?

What is physical fitness all about? What kinds of changes can be expected? How long does it take? What kinds of exercise should be performed to achieve fitness? How often? When? These and other questions must be answered, and the answers must be applied before the desired results can be achieved.

Similarly, how is weight loss accomplished? How long does it take? Can it be harmful? What is a "correct" weight, and how is it determined? To lose weight permanently, people must understand and apply basic physiological and nutritional facts.

Exercise physiologists and doctors interested in sports medicine and nutrition are working on the answers, but too often this information is published only in professional journals that are read by other experts and not by the general public. The general public gleans its information from nonprofessionals or from those interested in physical fitness from only a commercial standpoint.

Before we continue, two terms need to be explained: *total fitness* and *physical fitness*. Total fitness is usually considered to include physical, mental, emotional, social, medical, and nutritional fitness. The symbol of the YMCA depicts a triangle with the sides representing mental, spiritual, and physical fitness. Although each element of total fitness is important, this book deals mainly with physical fitness. Physical fitness is the part of total fitness that is concerned with the effects of exercise on the body and with the body's functions. It is influenced by nutrition, so this book reflects an interest in and concern with nutrition, diet, weight control, and body composition.

Components of Physical Fitness

The easiest way to define physical fitness is to subdivide it into its component parts. Early investigators tried to express physical fitness as a single score, often based primarily on strength tests. For instance, the Physical Fitness Index, as expressed in a single numerical score, was an expression of a person's physical fitness level. More recently, however, researchers have proposed that physical fitness is a profile of a number of different components. It is possible to score high in one component and low in another. The chief components are cardiorespiratory fitness, muscular strength and endurance, and flexibility. Other components often mentioned are agility, balance, reaction time, coordination, power, and speed; however, these are more commonly classified as motor fitness components.

Cardiorespiratory Fitness

Sometimes referred to as endurance or stamina, cardiorespiratory fitness denotes fitness of the heart and circulatory system. The popular term is *aerobics* or *aerobic power*. Other terms used in discussions of cardiorespiratory fitness are *oxygen uptake*, *maximum oxygen uptake*, *oxygen transportation*, *METs*, *target heart rate*, and *maximum heart rate*. (Exercise leaders should be familiar with these terms and their definitions.) Aerobic activities improve the transportation of oxygen through the blood to the working muscles by improving the efficiency of the heart, which pumps the blood; the lungs, where the blood picks up the oxygen; and the unloading of oxygen at the tissue level. Although the development of cardiorespiratory fitness will be discussed in detail later, in general it is developed through prolonged activity that demands that the blood transport large amounts of oxygen to the tissues. Excellent cardiorespiratory fitness activities include running, swimming, cycling, and cross-country skiing.

Muscular Strength and Endurance

Muscular strength is the ability to exert force through the recruitment of the maximum possible number of muscle fibers (cells) to overcome a resistance. The more muscle fibers that can be brought into action, the greater the strength. Progressively increasing the amount of resistance a muscle must overcome will train the muscle and the neural input to the muscle to work more efficiently, resulting in the use of more fibers. Strength is important, as all movement requires muscles. In addition, skeletal muscle strains and pulls can often be traced to poor muscular fitness and/or muscle-group imbalances.

Muscular endurance is the ability of a muscle to exercise for an extended period of time without undue fatigue. Unlike strength, muscular endurance is not measured by one maximum contraction but rather by multiple submaximal contractions. It is usually measured by the number of repetitions that can be done against a resistance, such as the number of push-ups, sit-ups, or curls that can be performed.

Flexibility

Flexibility is an attribute of joints and muscles. It is the ability of the muscles surrounding the joint to allow the joint its full range of motion. Flexibility exercises involve stretching the muscles rather than working against resistance. Athletes and people involved in exercise programs should spend time before and after the muscular and cardiorespiratory parts of the program doing flexibility exercises.

Attaining Physical Fitness

To be totally physically fit, an individual should attain more than an average level of fitness in each of the mentioned components. A good physical fitness program will include activities aimed at improving each component. Fortunately, more than one component can be developed by a single activity.

Appearance alone will not tell if someone is physically fit. A man may be lean, broad-shouldered, and small-waisted and still not be fit. Even a person whose job requires physical labor and who has developed strength may not be fit. Some time ago, fitness tests given to both manual laborers and office workers showed that although manual laborers were usually stronger, they were no more cardiorespiratorially fit than were office workers. Physiologists immediately interpreted these facts to mean that weightlifters and bodybuilders were unfit except for strength. As a consequence, many physical educators did not consider bodybuilders to be athletes. This attitude motivated considerable interest in studying ''weight'' athletes. Subsequent studies showed that these athletes had excellent flexibility, agility, speed, power, and balance as well as strength.

The major weakness among most of them was aerobic power, or cardiorespiratory fitness. Many bodybuilders responded to this criticism by adding running to their exercise routines, not necessarily to increase their weightlifting ability, but to improve their total physical fitness, especially their cardiorespiratory endurance. Today in YMCAs, private gyms, or anywhere that bodybuilders work out, jogging and other cardiorespiratory activities are commonplace.

With the dawn of the running boom, a problem of unbalanced physical fitness has developed again. Because of the tremendous interest in aerobic exercise and its possible effect in preventing heart disease, running has become extremely popular as a means of exercising the heart, lungs, and circulation. Although it is an excellent cardiorespiratory activity, one type of exercise alone does not make a person physically fit. The common and familiar story is that many runners want only to run; they seldom want to participate in a calisthenics or weight-training program. Running is an effective form of exercise, but it does nothing for the muscles of the arms, chest, back, or abdomen. Because running stresses the joints, there is a need for strong musculature. Road races and marathons may be a runner's goals, but they are not necessarily the goal of the national programs; total physical fitness is. Running and jogging are good means to achieving this goal, as is swimming; however, they all should be supplemented with strength and flexibility exercises.

Some people become extremely biased about their particular type of exercise and expect it to be the complete answer to physical fitness. Criticizing their activity is tantamount to criticizing their favorite political candidate. Advocates of yoga, belly dancing, skating, handball, weightlifting, jogging, or swimming all want to believe that their activity is the most complete and most desirable for attaining physical fitness. Yoga enthusiasts, for example, may interpret criticism of the limitations of yoga as meaning that yoga has no value. Yoga is excellent for relaxation, flexibility, agility, grace, strength, and coordination; however, it does little for cardiorespiratory endurance.

Because physical fitness is made up of various components, a test battery is required. That is why the national YMCA physical fitness evaluation is a battery of individual test items designed to measure cardiorespiratory endurance, muscular strength and endurance, flexibility, and body composition (see chapter 4).

EXERCISE PROGRAM PLANNING

One of the most difficult concepts to grasp is the value of each physical activity to the development of overall physical fitness. What is good exercise? How can a program be planned around it?

Recreational Sport and Fitness

There is a significant difference between playing a sport competitively, especially at a high level, and playing a sport recreationally. Handball, tennis, racquetball, swimming, and other sports require a high degree of physical fitness and also produce fitness when performed in a highly competitive situation. The same activities, however, performed recreationally, may require only a low level of fitness and will do nothing to increase fitness levels.

Recreational games and sports are very desirable and valuable, but the majority of recreational sports participants do not develop physical fitness. However, if participants are physically fit, their fitness will often enable them to play for extended periods of time without undue fatigue. This follows the saying, "You should get into shape to play sports, not play sports to get into shape."

Although most recreational activities do little to improve fitness, some can when performed properly. For instance, walking is an excellent activity for older persons or for those with lower aerobic capacity. But can a 40-year-old person in reasonably good physical condition develop cardiorespiratory fitness from walking? Yes, if the individual walks briskly and increases the heart rate to the proper level of training. Should that person run? Not necessarily. Too many people feel that running is the only mode of exercise that produces effective training; this is not true. Any activity that produces a sustained increase in heart rate for the appropriate duration, done regularly, will produce a training effect.

Principles of Training

Several principles of training should be considered when planning an exercise program.

Specificity, Overload, and Progression (SOP)

The principles of specificity, overload, and progression should become the standard operating procedure for class leaders when recommending exercise. The principle of specificity says that exercises must be done that specifically utilize a certain muscle if that muscle is to become stronger. Thus, any exercise program should include a variety of exercises utilizing all major parts of the body. The principle of overload emphasizes that the body is a very adaptable mechanism; as work is presented to the body it adapts to that work and more work can be done. This means that, although at the beginning of a program the amount of work undertaken should not be strenuous, the workload should be increased gradually over time. The amount of increased work is decided by adaptation; each type of exercise is different, and the amount of work for each may be increased at different rates. Finally, the principle of progression means that to promote physical fitness it is necessary to do more work each week than was done the week before. At each level of work adaptation takes place; progress may be slow, but steadily the body becomes more efficient and capable of more work.

Retrogression

Retrogression is the plateauing of improvement that often occurs after a few weeks of exercise. Being aware of this phenomenon may avoid discouragement and disappointment. During the first few weeks of exercise great strides are made, and improvement is noticeable and satisfactory. After a few weeks (the time will vary) progress appears to stop, and a participant may feel that there is no additional improvement. Retrogression is normal and common. Because of the lack of understanding of this phenomenon and the resulting frustration and disappointment, many home programs are stopped at this point. But, if the program is continued, progression will again occur.

Training Specificity

Training is very specific; this means that specific areas of fitness are developed by participation in each particular sport. The type of program discussed in this chapter will build general overall physical fitness as a solid foundation for the more specific fitness capabilities needed for specific activities.

Frequency, Intensity, and Time (FIT)

Frequency, intensity, and time are three principles involved in all progressive exercise programs. How often, how long, and how hard should a participant exercise? A summary of many studies indicates that 3 to 4 days per week is the minimum number of times that exercise should occur. Exercise 5 or 6 days a week is better, but changes will occur with only three times per week. Intensity is addressed in a later section of this chapter, ''Control of Exercise Intensity,'' and time is discussed next.

Session Time Allotment

Thirty minutes well spent is a minimum per session; 45 minutes is better. As shown in Figure 5-1, the time is used differently at the beginning of the sessions than it is toward the end.

Early in a starter fitness program more time is devoted to warm-up and cool-down and less to strength and flexibility exercises and cardiorespiratory training. Because participants are learning the correct form and sequence for routines and are less fit, there is considerable time between exercises, and exercises are done slowly with few repetitions. Each exercise is done for a set period of time rather than for a certain number of repetitions (e.g., abdominal work for 30 seconds to 1 minute).

As the program progresses, the time allotted for warm-up and cool-down decreases (see Fig. 5-1). However, the improved condition of the participants permits exercise at a faster pace. By the final weeks of the class, a 45-minute program can be divided as follows:

10 minutes—*warm-up: rhythmic exercises, low intensity, stretching and increasing flexibility/range of movement; flexibility exercises*
10 minutes—*strength and muscular endurance exercises: calisthenics, weightlifting*
20 minutes—*cardiorespiratory exercises: jogging, swimming, cycling*
5 minutes—*cool down: walking, stretching, relaxing*

45 minutes—total

As the participants adapt and progress, more of the 45-minute period is used until the time is being utilized to the maximum; no more miles can be jogged or no more calisthenic repetitions can be performed because there is no more time. However, overload can be realized by increasing the intensity, that is, by moving a little faster or increasing the resistance.

When the 45 minutes have been filled with exercise done at 85% of maximum, a certain level of fitness will have been reached and no more progress will occur. The program then will change from a fitness-producing program to a fitness-maintenance program.

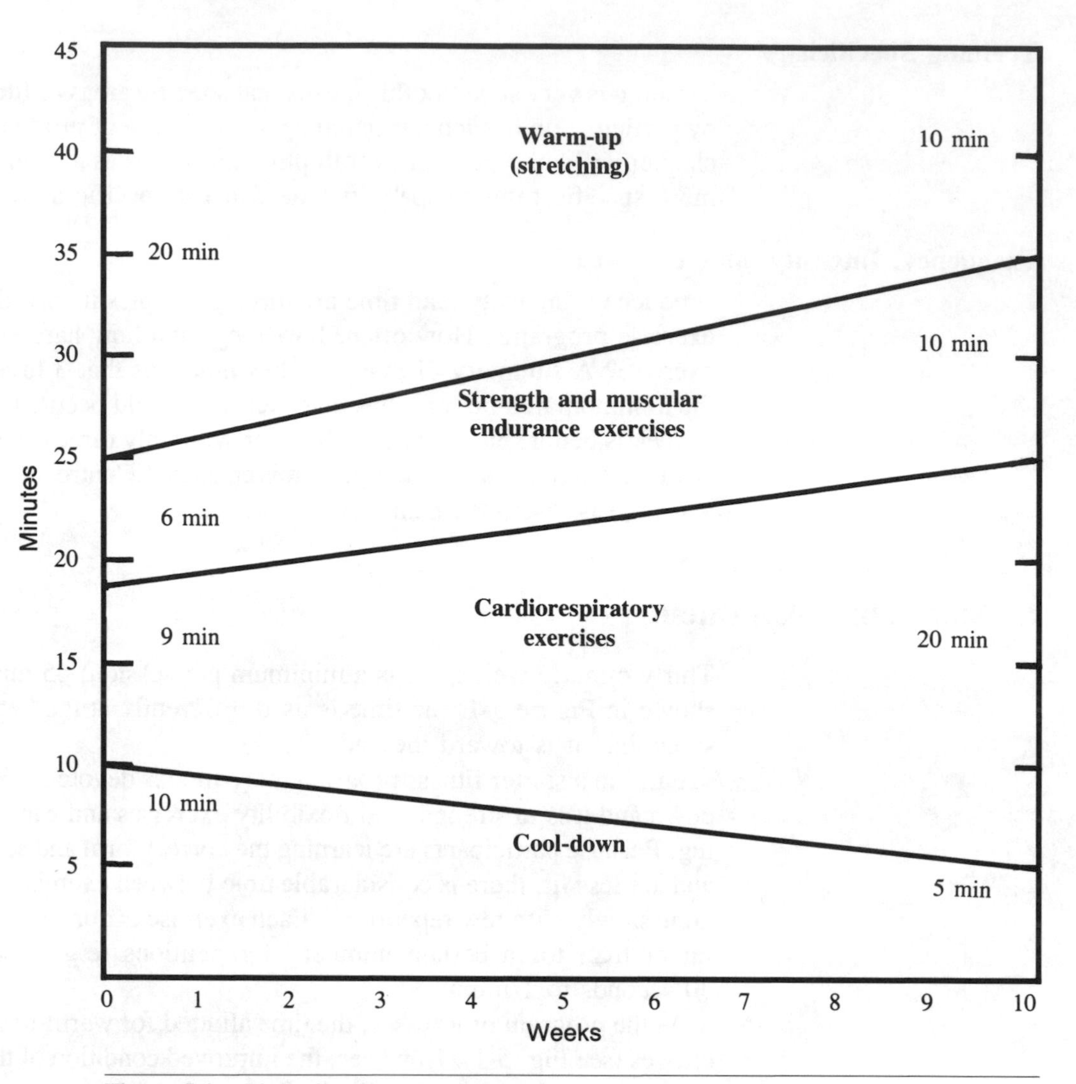

Figure 5-1. Time allotments for main parts of exercise session.

Weekly Progression

The intensity of exercises and the number of repetitions will increase as a program progresses from week to week. There is no set progression; how much a class progresses is a function of the individuals in the class. Some classes have younger, fitter, or more faithful participants than have others or have participants who adapt to exercise more quickly. Everyone is different; not everyone progresses or adapts at the same rate. Each participant will respond to the exercise program in his or her own way. Participants should be encouraged to focus on the changes occurring in their own fitness level and not on the accomplishments of others.

By leading the class and observing and listening to participants, an instructor can determine the amount of weekly progression. There is nothing wrong with staying at a particular level for 2 or more weeks before progressing.

PRECAUTIONARY MEASURES

Before planning a specific exercise program for a particular group of participants, the instructor should be aware of some precautionary measures related to all exercise programs.

Participants' Ability to Begin Exercise

Participants should have a good medical evaluation by a physician and a physical fitness evaluation before they begin any exercise program (see chapter 4). Prior to the first class meeting, results of tests and medical history forms should be reviewed. Those who are over 60 years old, are obese, or have high blood pressure or orthopedic problems should be carefully evaluated before they are allowed to participate in the regular fitness program. A final review of medical history forms will reconfirm that participants have no previously overlooked conditions that would contraindicate exercise. The instructor should be aware of any special needs that individuals may have.

When physical fitness tests cannot be administered prior to starting exercise, walking instead of jogging should be used as the cardiovascular endurance exercise until it is clear that all participants are able to respond favorably to the increased physical activity. Individuals scoring very poorly on the bicycle test or step test may be required to participate in a preliminary walking program to develop a minimum fitness level before entering a regular class. Anyone who shows excessive breathing and heart-rate response to the regular exercises is a potential candidate for such preconditioning activities.

A practical hint is to develop a confidential list based on participants' medical clearance forms that identifies persons at risk. A dot may be placed next to those participants' names on the attendance sheet, and those people should receive particularly close attention.

Control of Exercise Intensity

Exercise leaders must keep the intensity of the workout within the capacities of individual participants. The most convenient way of doing this for jogging and other cardiorespiratory activities is to teach participants how to take their pulse rates immediately after exercise and to use them as a guide. Heart rates taken during the first 15 seconds following exercise are quite close to the exercise value. An acceptable target heart rate is between 65% and 85% of the predicted maximum heart rate estimated for a person's age (220 minus age). That is equivalent to an energy expenditure of approximately 50% of the maximum oxygen intake. When a person first enters a fitness program the target heart rate should be 65% of the predicted maximum heart rate. After adequate progression and time this target heart rate can be increased to 75% and then to 85% if it can be tolerated. As heart rate decreases with age, this value becomes lower with passing years. Table 5-1 is a scale of estimated heart rates that may be used.

Table 5-1 Estimated Target Heart Rates

Age	Predicted max HR	Target heart rate 65%	75%	85%
20-29	191-200	124-130	143-150	162-170
30-39	181-190	118-123	136-142	154-161
40-49	171-180	111-117	129-135	145-153
50-59	161-170	105-110	121-128	137-144

Hypertension medications such as beta blockers may affect the heart rate. For participants using such medication, consult with the medical advisory committee and consider using perceived exertion as an indicator of intensity. Perceived exertion simply means that an individual who feels (perceives) he or she is working hard probably is (see question 87 in chapter 3).

The instructor should familiarize participants with warning signs of overexertion such as excessive heart rate, heavy breathing, pale skin, and flushing. Participants exhibiting these signs should exercise at a reduced level until they develop the capacity to handle more intense exercise. A brisk walking or bicycle ergometer program may be suggested.

Danger Signs

Although the signs just mentioned indicate a need for modifying a participant's activities, they are not signs of imminent danger. The signs that do indicate danger and signal that exercise must be stopped immediately are as follows:

- Labored breathing (difficult breathing, not the deep breathing normally associated with exercise)
- Loss of coordination
- Dizziness
- Tightness in chest

If any of these signs occur, exercise should not be continued until medical advice is obtained.

Watch particularly carefully when exercising under extremely hot conditions. Heat stress can be very dangerous and can occur in the gymnasium as well as in the sun. Review the guidelines presented in chapter 3.

Leader's Responsibility

Desirable characteristics and training of the exercise leader are discussed in chapter 2; however, there are several responsibilities of the class leader that are directly related to conducting the exercise program. The class leader needs to remember that it is not his or her workout that is important but rather that of the class members. The class leader should always

- be alert for signs of too fast a pace;
- watch for signs of overexertion;

- caution participants to resist competitive urges, which lead to overstress;
- try to maintain a friendly, fun climate for the class;
- adjust the workout to accommodate daily and seasonal differences in temperature and humidity; and
- maintain daily records on attendance.

The leader is responsible for keeping records on participants' progress. Ultimately it is the leader's judgment as to the ability of the individuals in the class to advance from one level to the next. A leader should know the class and be responsible for it.

SESSION GUIDELINES

An exercise session should consist of four basic parts—warm-up, muscular strength and endurance exercises, cardiorespiratory work, and cool-down. Everyone should exercise a minimum of 40 to 60 minutes three to four times per week (see chapter 3, question 85).

A 10-week exercise progression is illustrated in Table 5-2. Exercises should be selected to develop strength and muscular endurance, flexibility, and cardiorespiratory endurance. Again, during the early weeks of the program there is a greater amount of time devoted to warm-up than there is later; the converse is true for cardiorespiratory endurance. This is done to allow for the generally poor condition of new participants. During the first weeks, warm-up exercises are stressful enough to produce a training effect.

Table 5-2 Sample Weekly Time Progressions for Beginner's Program

		Muscular strength and endurance (min)					Cardiorespiratory (min)		
Week	Warm-up (min)	Back	Abdomen	Legs	Shoulders and arms	Total	Run/walk sets	Total	Cool-down (min)
1	20	1	2	1	3	6	4 run/walk	9	10
2	18	1	2	2	3	8	4 run/walk	9	10
3	18	1	2	2	3	8	4 run/walk	9	10
4	16	1	2	2	3	8	6 run/walk	12	9
5	16	1	2	2	3	8	2-4 run/1 walk	12	9
6	15	1	2	3	3	9	2-4 run/1 walk	12	9
7	14	1	3	3	3	10	3-4 run/1 walk	16	5
8	13	1	3	3	3	10	3-4 run/1 walk	16	6
9	11	1	3	3	3	10	3-5 run/1 walk	18	6
10	10	1	3	3	3	10	3-6 run/1 walk	20	5

Note. Total session lasts 45 min.

Strength and muscle endurance exercises usually follow the warm-up period. Additional stretching exercises are included within the strength and endurance exercise time allotment.

Whenever possible, include education on fitness topics for participants. An easy way to do this is to give 5 to 10 minute minilectures at the beginning or end of class, even during warm-up or cool-down. Outlines for a series of 20 minilectures appear in *Health Enhancement for America's Work Force—Program Guide* (YMCA of the USA, 1987).

The following guidelines for planning the four main parts of an exercise program should be adhered to for any exercise plan.

Warm-Up

Purpose: The purpose of the warm-up period is to prepare the body for the work to come.

Guidelines for Planning Warm-Up

1. Gradually increase the intensity of exercise as the warm-up progresses.
2. Include exercises that gently stretch the muscles and joints through their full range of motion. Resistance should not be used.
3. Choose warm-up exercises that are rhythmic in nature and order them in a sequence planned to flow naturally from one exercise to another.
4. Perform different exercises on different days; variety makes warm-ups more enjoyable and interesting.
5. Do not spend more than 20 minutes on warm-up initially. The amount of time spent will necessarily decrease as participants' fitness improves and other periods take more time.
6. Include both stretching exercises and exercises that increase the activity of the heart and circulatory system. Some instructors like to separate warm-up and stretching.

Suitable Exercises for Warm-Up

All body segments should be exercised and stretched in a warm-up routine. Exercises that include the following movements should be used. A single exercise may incorporate several of these movements.

- Flexion, extension, and rotation of the neck
- Flexion, extension, rotation, and circumduction of the shoulder joints
- Flexion, extension, slight rotation, and circumduction of the trunk
- Flexion, extension, abduction, and circumduction of the hip joints (especially stretch the hamstrings)
- Flexion and extension of the knees
- Plantar flexion and dorsiflexion of the ankles (especially stretch the calves)

Muscular Strength and Endurance Training

Purpose: To provide resistance to each major muscle group to improve the strength of these muscles.

Guidelines for Planning Muscular Strength and Endurance Training

1. Include exercises for all major joint movements of the different body segments.
2. Do not develop undue circulatory resistance. Avoid Valsalva maneuvers (see chapter 3). It is better to do resistance exercises in sets rather than

continuously to exhaustion. For example, if the goal is to do 10 push-ups in a moderately conditioned group, it is better to do two sets of 5 rather than one set of 10.
3. Do not do free-swinging exercises against fixed joints, as this strains muscles, tendons, and ligaments. For example, do not force toe touching by bouncing with the knees locked.
4. Maintain a high level of activity without creating local fatigue by shifting exercises from muscle group to muscle group. This means, for example, not doing more than two consecutive abdominal exercises.
5. Plan the exercise sequence so there is movement from exercise to exercise with minimum hesitation. Use a written outline of the exercise routine if necessary or post the routine in large print (perhaps on a blackboard) so that the class also knows the day's sequence of exercise.
6. Encourage participants to work at their own rate. Do *not* insist that all class members keep up with the group.
7. Emphasize using the full range of motion for all exercises.

Suitable Exercises for Muscular Strength and Endurance Training

The following is a list of commonly used calisthenics and the muscle groups involved. Each exercise is illustrated by one or more photographs. Other calisthenics may be used, and descriptions of these exercises are readily available. Small classes may decide to use weights for strength development, which is an excellent idea but usually not practical in large-class situations.

- Push-up—posterior arms, chest, shoulders (Figs. 5-2 and 5-3)
- Straddle chin—anterior arms, chest (Fig. 5-4)
- Chest raise—back, buttocks, posterior thighs (Fig. 5-5) (Do not try to raise too high or jerk. Do it slowly.)
- Bench step—thighs, buttocks, calves (Fig. 5-6) (For a complete sequence of the bench step see Figure 4-27.)
- Lateral leg raise—lateral thighs (Fig. 5-7)
- Half squat—anterior thighs, calves (Fig. 5-8)
- Bent-knee sit-up—abdominals (Fig. 5-9)
- Abdominal crunch—abdominals (Fig. 5-10)
- Kneel-lean—posterior thighs (Fig. 5-11)
- Ab/ad—inside/outside thighs (Fig. 5-12)

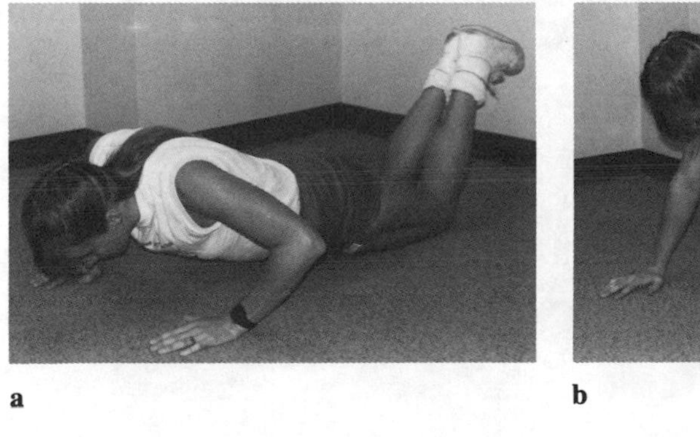
a

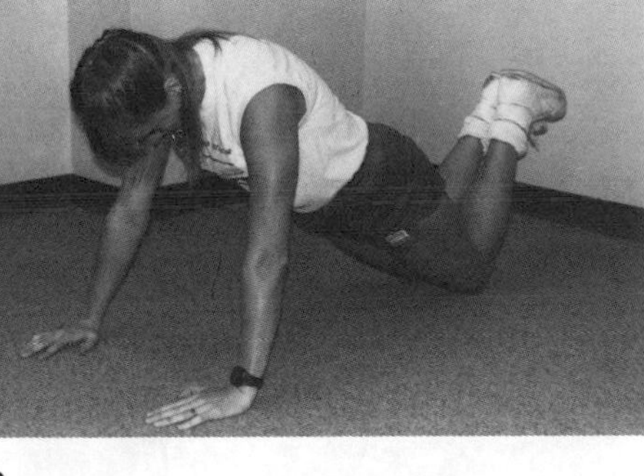
b

Figure 5-2. Bent-knee push-up. (a) Down position; (b) up position.

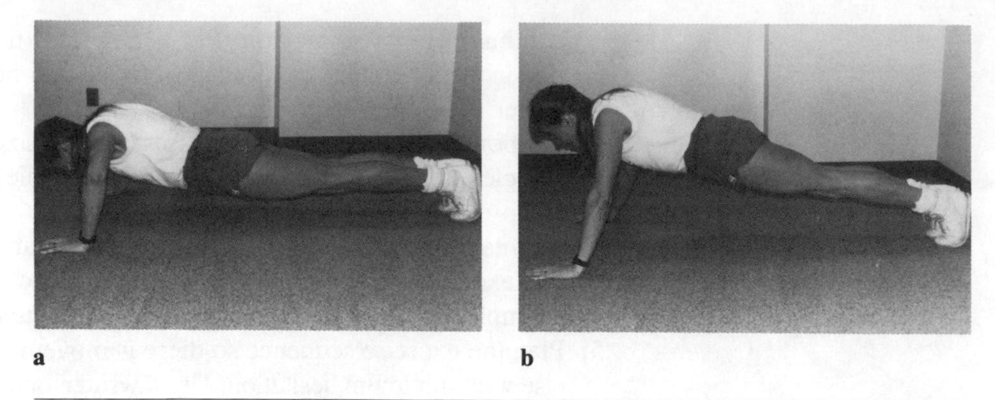

a b

Figure 5-3. Straight-legged push-up. (a) Down position; (b) up position.

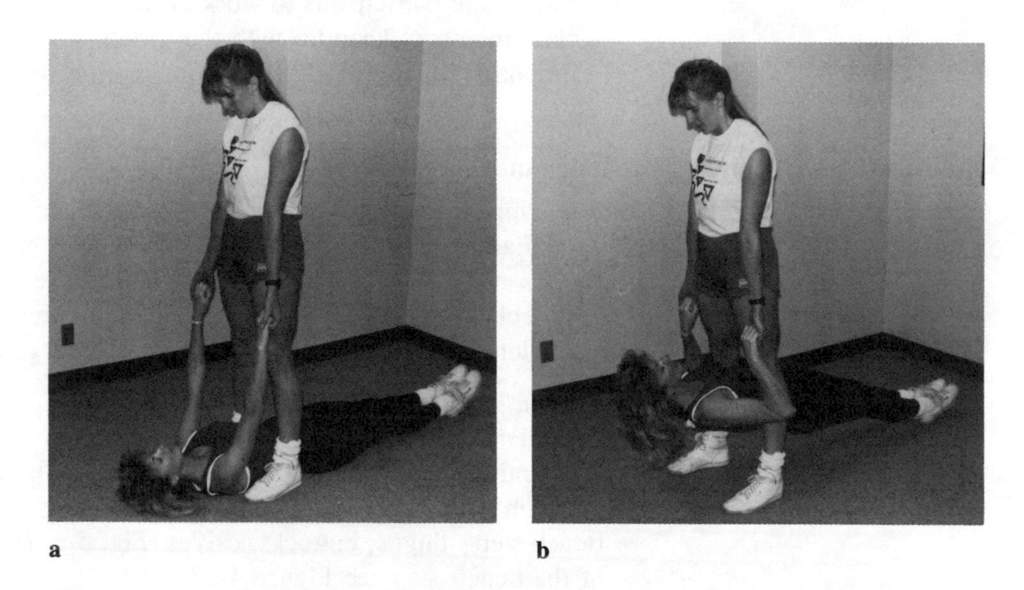

a b

Figure 5-4. Straddle chin. (a) Down position; (b) up position.

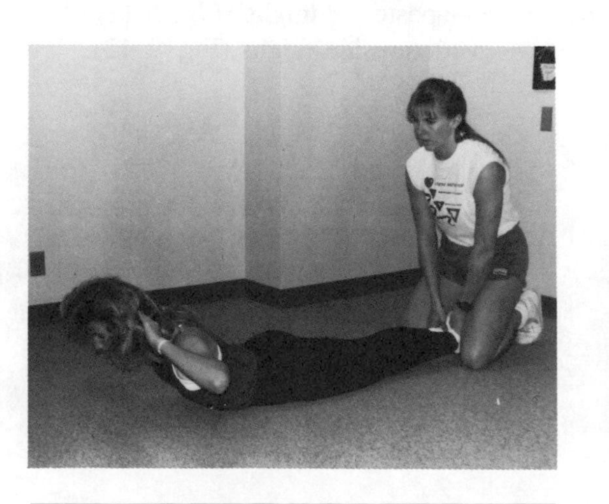

Figure 5-5. Chest raise.

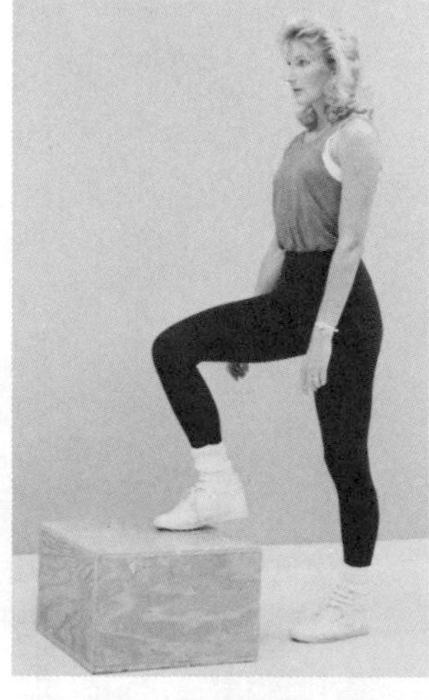

Figure 5-6. Bench step.

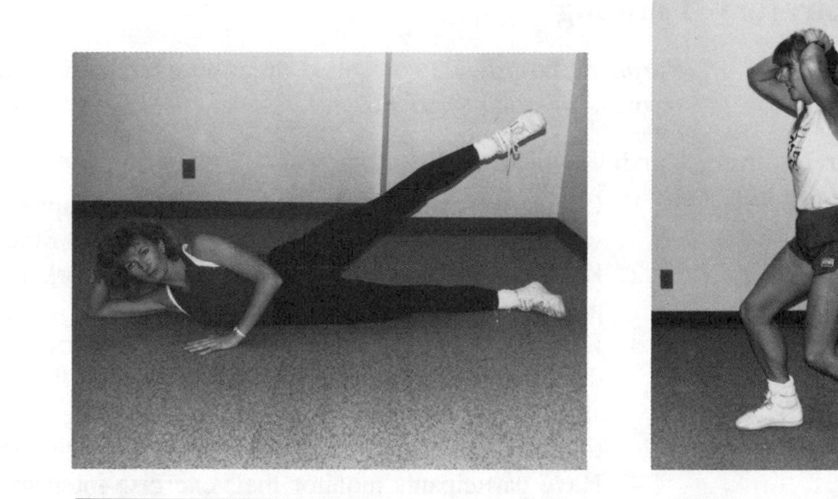

Figure 5-7. Lateral leg raise.

Figure 5-8. Half squat.

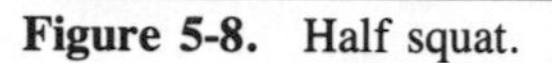

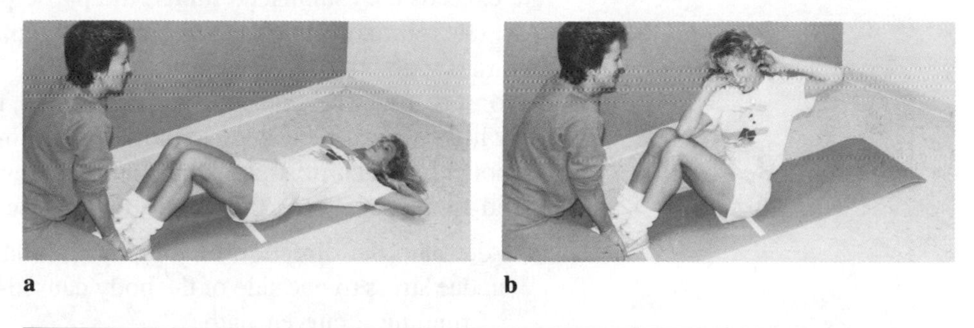

a b

Figure 5-9. Bent-knee sit-up. (a) Down position; (b) up position.

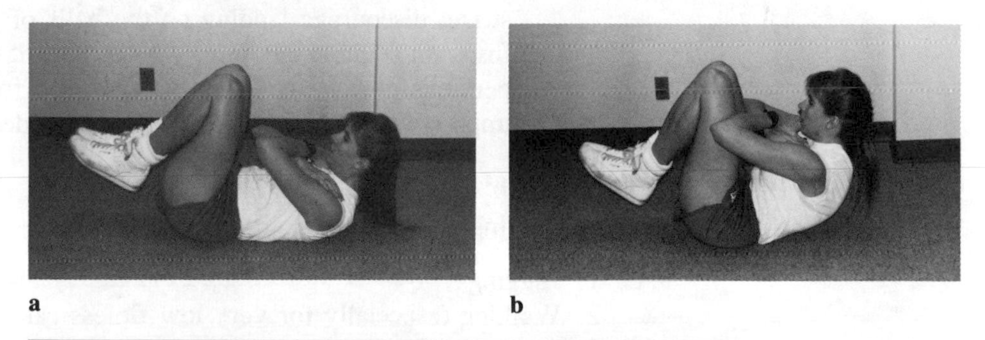

a b

Figure 5-10. Abdominal crunch. (a) Down position; (b) up position.

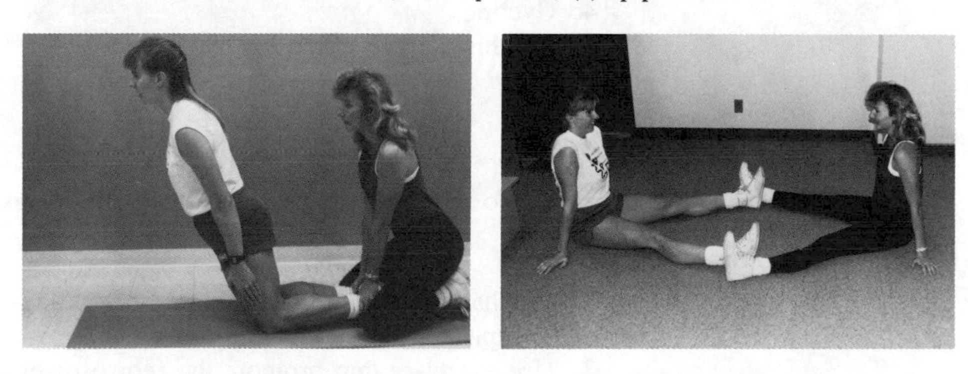

Figure 5-11. Kneel-lean.

Figure 5-12. Ab/ad.

Cardiorespiratory Training

Purpose: To provide controlled duration exercise in order to induce cardiorespiratory training effects.

Guidelines for Planning Cardiorespiratory Training

1. Choose a training program that is readily adaptable to individual needs while still permitting the group approach to fitness.
2. Keep the interval principle—alternation of work and rest—in mind when planning program progression.
3. For beginner's programs, restrict training progression to increasing the duration of exercise intervals while keeping the exercise intensity constant. In advanced programs (beyond intermediate) both exercise duration and intensity may be varied to produce the desired training effect.
4. Have participants monitor their exercise intensity individually. Heart-rate monitoring can be used for this purpose. When the exercise heart rate exceeds the established limits, the participant should walk until the heart rate returns to its normal limits. This applies to any form of cardiorespiratory activity.
5. Be conservative when working with untrained, middle-aged participants. Very little exercise is needed to induce a training response in this group.
6. Do not permit a competitive atmosphere to develop among participants.
7. Avoid running patterns that might be harmful:
   a. Alternate the direction of jogging around a gym track to prevent undue stress to one side of the body caused by the mechanical effects of running a curved path.
   b. Encourage participants to jog with either a heel-toe or a flat foot-strike; discourage landing on the balls of the feet or the toes.
   c. Insist on suitable clothing. Do not permit rubberized or other impervious gear in the gymnasium. Good footwear is of the utmost importance if leg soreness is to be avoided.

Suitable Exercises for Cardiorespiratory Training

The following are suitable exercises:

1. Jogging
2. Walking (especially for very low fitness categories)
3. Swimming
4. Cycling
5. Rhythmic exercise to music

Cool-Down

Purpose: To return the body gradually to the nonexercising state.

Guidelines for Planning Cool-Down

1. Emphasize relaxing exercise.
2. Complete the period in 5 to 10 minutes.
3. Use exercises that promote the return of blood to the heart from the extremities.

4. Make sure that participants' heart rates show adequate recovery by the end of the cool-down period, depending on their fitness levels (less than 100 to 110 bpm).

Suitable Exercises for Cool-Down

The following are suitable exercises. They should be performed in a relaxed fashion.

1. Mild jogging and walking
2. Hands-over-head stretch side to side
3. Front-crawl motion of arms while standing or walking
4. Mild stretching exercises done on the floor (seated, prone, and/or supine)

COMMENTS FROM SUCCESSFUL EXERCISE LEADERS

To end this chapter, here is a potpourri of comments from experienced leaders about ways to lead exercise classes successfully:

- Get to know the names and interests of class members.
- Develop a "buddy system" for new members; make them feel at home through personal contact with you and other class members.
- Be sure to talk to members, both old and new; let them know that you are interested in them and show that interest.
- Keep the class fun. The class must be enjoyable.
- Try to get all members to relax completely before starting the warm-up and again after cool-down.
- Work some basic back-flexibility exercises into the warm-up period.
- Work at developing class leadership abilities and skills. Watch other leaders and attend training sessions.
- Maintain interest; keep attendance up with special incentives.
- Many members drop out because they are overworked (too tired and too sore). Plan a conservative progression so that participants can adapt successfully.
- Be aware of the difficulties of leading a class with members of mixed abilities and different levels of fitness.
- Promote the program (see chapter 2).
- Review your own knowledge about physical fitness, exercise, and diet regularly. This review should include new data, methods, and beliefs and should reinforce the concept that the professional physical educator is not an exercise faddist but rather an educated leader.
- Call any participant who has missed 3 days in a row and invite him or her back.

As an aid to teaching fitness classes, you may want to copy the following pages. They include a table of estimated heart-rate ranges, a chart showing the relative length of different parts of the workout, and spaces for recording attendance and notes.

Target Heart Rate Ranges

Age	Predicted max HR	Target heart rate 65%	75%	85%
20-29	191-200	124-130	143-150	162-170
30-39	181-190	118-123	136-142	154-161
40-49	171-180	111-117	129-135	145-153
50-59	161-170	105-110	121-128	137-144

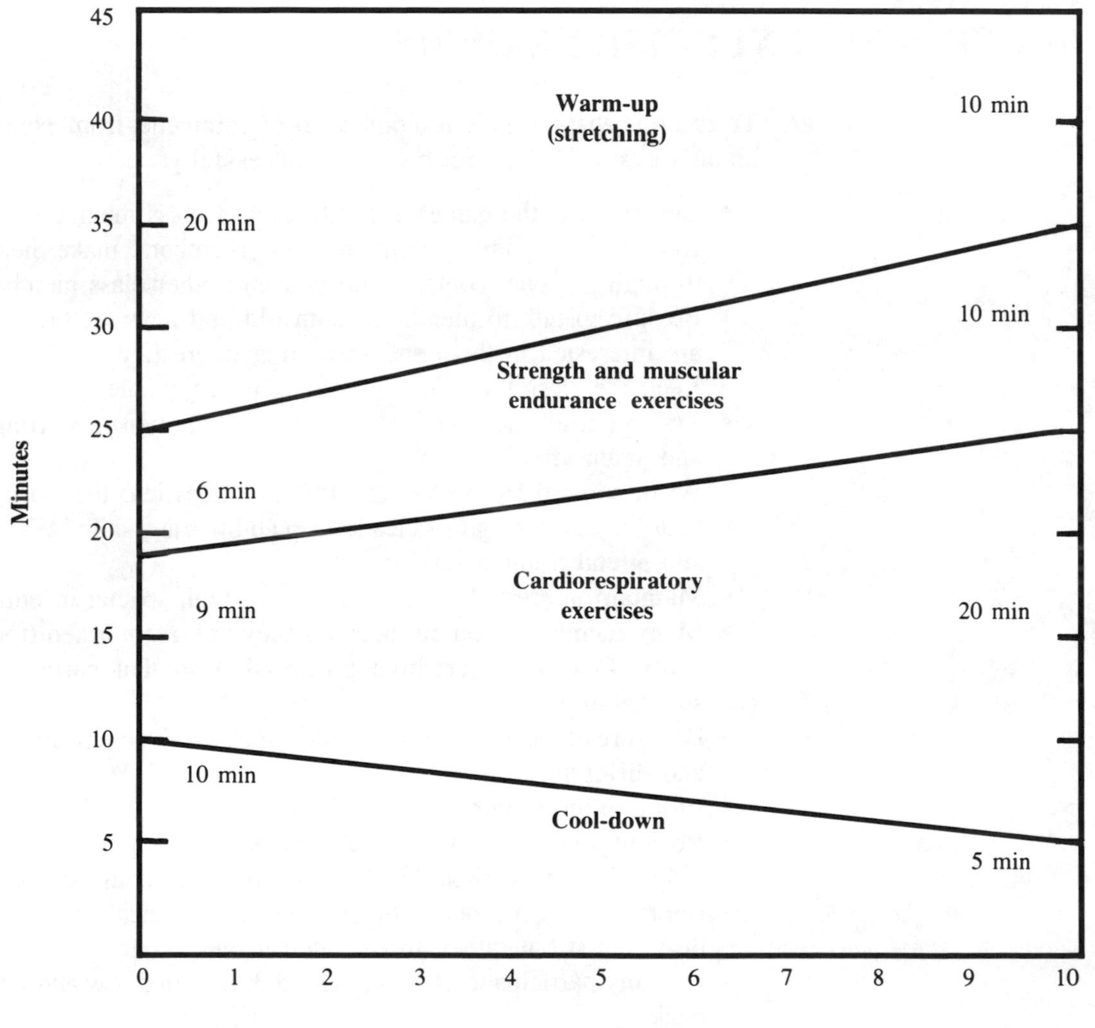

Attendance

Date										
Name										

Notes

Physical Fitness and Health Enhancement Program Resources

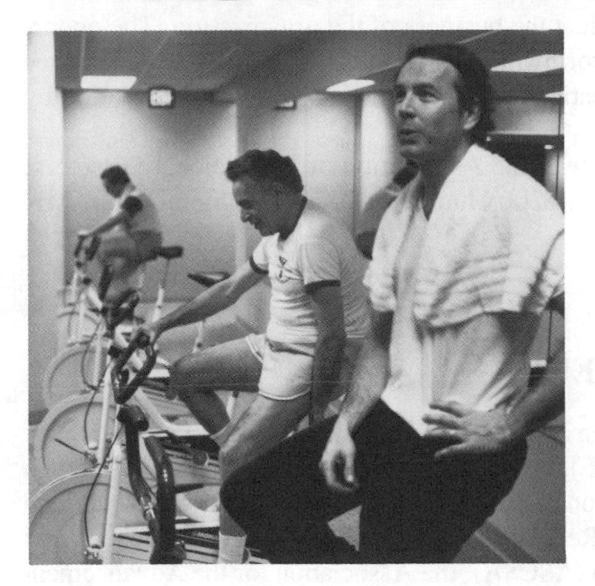

Chapter 6

The purpose of this chapter is to provide professional physical fitness leaders with sources for fitness information and leadership and program ideas. Such sources include organizations, books, and other materials. These resources will help leaders become more knowledgeable about physical fitness and perform their administrative and program duties more efficiently.

PROFESSIONAL ORGANIZATIONS

A resource overlooked by many physical fitness leaders is membership in professional organizations. Not only do these groups provide related materials and information, but important professional contacts may be made at their state, regional, and national conferences. Thus, when leaders join, they should become involved in the organizations' activities.

Related organizations are described here, and addresses are listed for additional information.

National YMCA Physical Education Society

The National YMCA Physical Education Society is a section of the Association of Professional Directors of the YMCA of the USA. Professional physical educators employed by YMCAs are eligible for membership. Its purpose is to unite the professional directors of physical education within the YMCA, thus giving them a unified voice at the national level.

The society provides many services. Conferences at the local, district, and national levels are held to provide training and the general dissemination of information, as well as to conduct the business of the organization. The opportunity for the recognition of worthwhile research is also available; acceptance of such work provides certification as a Directorate of Physical Education by the national society.

For further information, write to the Association of Professional Directors, Commerce Building, Suite 111, 8200 Humboldt Avenue, Bloomington, MN 55431.

American Alliance for Health, Physical Education, Recreation and Dance (AAHPERD)

AAHPERD is made up of seven associations: the National Association of Sport and Physical Education (NASPE), the National Association for Girls and Women in Sport (NAGWS), the National Dance Association (NDA), the American Association for Leisure and Recreation (AALR), the American School and Community Safety Association (ASCSA), the Association for the Advancement of Health Education (AAHE), and the Association for Research, Administration, Professional Councils and Societies (ARAPCS). AAHPERD conducts state, regional, and national conferences that almost always have presentations on physical fitness and related research. Many pertinent publications are also available. Smaller groups that are especially of interest to people working in physical fitness are the Physical Fitness Council of ARAPCS, the Physiology of Exercise Academy of NASPE, and the Research Consortium, which deals with research on physical fitness.

For further information, write to the American Alliance for Health, Physical Education, Recreation and Dance, 1900 Association Drive, Reston, VA 22091.

American College of Sports Medicine (ACSM)

ACSM is the foremost organization in the sport sciences today. Not only does ACSM promote research, it also sponsors regional and national meetings, conferences, and educational programs. The organization edits and publishes journals and other materials and has certification procedures to qualify physical fitness personnel in two tracks: the preventive track and the rehabilitative track. The preventive track includes certification as an exercise leader, a health/fitness instructor, or a health/fitness director. The rehabilitative track includes certification as an exercise test technologist, an exercise specialist, or an exercise program director.

The membership of ACSM is quite diverse. It includes not only physicians, exercise physiologists, and exercise biochemists but also athletic trainers, high school physical educators, physical fitness leaders, and others whose work is more applied than theoretical.

For further information, write to the American College of Sports Medicine, P.O. Box 1440, Indianapolis, IN 46206-1440.

Association for Fitness in Business (AFB)

The membership of AFB consists of professional members who are employed by companies or organizations to conduct physical fitness programs, general members who may be engaged in physical fitness programming outside business and industry, and student members. The first purpose of the organization is to provide support and assistance in the development of physical fitness programs in business and industry. Other purposes are to cooperate with other organizations that promote fitness, recommend qualifications and standards for professional personnel, encourage and support in-service training, stimulate research, serve as a clearinghouse for information, and develop materials for fitness programs in business and industry.

For further information, write to Association for Fitness in Business, 310 North Alabama, Suite A100, Indianapolis, IN 46204.

International Dance-Exercise Association (IDEA)

This group is the largest association for aerobics and dance-exercise professionals in the world. Individual and business memberships are available. The group provides its members with up-to-date information on exercise physiology, injury prevention, and nutrition and focuses on new ideas in choreography and music for use in classes. The organization publishes a magazine, *Dance Exercise Today*, as well as other exercise-related publications. Training events are held, some for certification, through the IDEA Foundation, which sets standards for training, administers certification exams, provides consumer education, and promotes research for the dance-exercise field. Other benefits include reduced-cost liability insurance and discounts on fitness products.

For further information, write to International Dance-Exercise Association, 6190 Cornerstone Court East, Suite 204, San Diego, CA 92121-3773.

A list of other organizations that can offer leaders information, help, and training follows.

Aerobics & Fitness Association of America
15250 Ventura Boulevard, Suite 310
Sherman Oaks, CA 91403

American Academy of Pediatrics
Box 927
141 NW Point Boulevard
Elk Grove Village, IL 60007

American Academy of Podiatric Sports Medicine
1729b Glastonberry Road
Potomac, MD 20854

American Cancer Society
90 Park Avenue
New York, NY 10016

American College of Cardiology
9111 Old Georgetown Road
Bethesda, MD 20814

American College of Preventive Medicine
1015 15th Street NW, Suite 403
Washington, DC 20005

American Dental Association
21 E. Chicago Avenue
Chicago, IL 60611

American Diabetes Association
1660 Duke Street
Alexandria, VA 22314

American Dietetic Association
208 S. LaSalle Street, Suite 1100
Chicago, IL 60604

American Heart Association
7320 Greenville Avenue
Dallas, TX 75231

American Hospital Association
36 S. Saute Street
Salt Lake City, UT 84111

American Medical Association
535 N. Dearborn Street
Chicago, IL 60610

American Medical Joggers Association
P.O. Box 4704
North Hollywood, CA 91607

American Osteopathic Academy of Sports Medicine
P.O. Box 623
Middleton, WI 53562

American Physical Therapy Association, Inc.
1111 N. Fairfax Street
Alexandria, VA 22314

American Public Health Association
1015 15th Street NW
Washington, DC 20005

American Red Cross
1730 E Street NW
Washington, DC 20006

American Running & Fitness Association
9310 Old Georgetown Road
Bethesda, MD 20814

American Society of Biomechanics
in Sports
2450 Lozana Road
Delmar, CA 92014

National Association of Governor's
Councils for Physical Fitness and Sport
PanAm Plaza
201 S. Capitol, Suite 440
Indianapolis, IN 46225

National Athletic Trainers Association
Philadelphia Eagles Veterans Stadium
Philadelphia, PA 19148

National Center for Health/Fitness
American University
3700 Nebraska Avenue NW
Washington, DC 20016

National Wellness Association
University of Wisconsin at Stevens Point
South Hall
Stevens Point, WI 54481

President's Council on Physical Fitness
& Sports
450 5th Street NW, Suite 7103
Washington, DC 20001

NATIONAL YMCA HEALTH ENHANCEMENT PROGRAM MATERIALS

The YMCA Program Store (P.O. Box 5076, Champaign, IL 61825-5076) has a variety of resources in the health enhancement field. Write or call 1-800-747-0089 for a catalog.

The YMCA of the USA has developed national fitness programs for the entire family. Each of the national programs has a number of resources designed for that program. They are listed below, under the name of the program.

Y's Way to Physical Fitness

- *Y's Way to Physical Fitness* (3rd ed.)
- *Y's Way to Physical Fitness Leader's Guide*
- *The Official YMCA Fitness Program*
- *How Fit Are You?* (videotape)

YMCA Programs for New Families

- *YMCA Programs for New Families*
- *Exercises for Baby & Me*

Y's Way to Water Exercise

- *Y's Way to Water Exercise*
- *Y's Way to Water Exercise Instructor's Guide*

Y's Way to Better Aerobics

- *Y's Way to Better Aerobics*
- *Y's Way to Better Aerobics Leader's Guide*

Y's Way to Weight Management

- *Y's Way to Weight Management*
- *Y's Way to Weight Management Log*
- *Y's Way to Weight Management Leader's Guide*
- *How Healthy Is Your Diet?* (videotape)

Y's Way to Stress Management

- *Kicking Your Stress Habits*
- *Y's Way to Stress Management Leader's Guide*
- *How Well Do You Manage Stress*? (videotape)

Y's Way to Strength Training

- *Building Strength at the YMCA*
- *Instructor Guide for the Y's Way to Strength Training*

The Y's Way to a Healthy Back

- *The Y's Way to a Healthy Back*
- *Say Goodbye to Back Pain* (videotape)

For YMCAs developing health enhancement programs for corporate clients, there is a two-volume set entitled *Health Enhancement for America's Work Force*, consisting of a *Program Guide* and an *Administrator's Guide*.

These are just some of the publications the YMCA Program Store has to offer; they have many more materials on exercise and fitness, as well as promotional materials for a number of the programs listed.

Sample Volunteer Job Descriptions

Appendix A

Job Title

Active older adults' fitness instructor

Responsible to

Mary Smith

Scheduled Times for This Position

10:00 a.m. to noon, Monday, Wednesday, Friday

Job Summary

The fitness instructor helps teach the basic guidelines of exercise, nutrition, and relaxation techniques to improve the quality of life for healthy participants.

Activities and Responsibilities

- Leads proper technique for warm-up, stretching, aerobic, cool-down, and relaxation exercises
- Is alert to overexertion, muscle injury, and other physical difficulties
- Arrives 10 minutes prior to class and stays 5 minutes afterward; is dependable and punctual
- Attends staff meetings when scheduled
- Calls program supervisor as soon as possible to notify in case of absence
- Gives 2 weeks' notice if withdrawal becomes necessary before end of commitment
- Ensures that exercise class contains all the necessary components as indicated in *Y's Way to Physical Fitness*

Needed Qualifications

- Is interested in learning new skills and ideas
- Enjoys people and has a positive attitude
- Has current CPR and first aid certification
- Wears proper exercise attire
- Is enthusiastic

Training and Job Preparation

- Observes and participates in class for a 6-week orientation period
- Attends YMCA fitness leader training
- Attends emergency procedures orientation

Supervision and Evaluation

- Program supervisor is available to discuss questions, progress, and difficulties.
- Program supervisor evaluates instructor every 6 weeks.
- Instructor evaluates the program and own experience on a regular basis.
- Recommendations are available on request.

Minimum Time Commitment

6 months

Job Title

Water Exercise Leader

Responsible to

Joe Johnson

Scheduled Times for This Position

6:00 p.m. to 8:00 p.m., Tuesday, Thursday

Job Summary

The volunteer leader conducts an aquatic exercise class implementing stretching, toning, and cardiovascular activities.

Activities and Responsibilities

- Develops a water exercise routine for adults
- Sets up equipment before class and puts it away after class
- If music is desired, arranges for its use
- Is constantly alert for overexertion, muscle injuries, and other physical difficulties
- Assists in maintaining a safe environment in the pool area
- Is available before and after class to answer questions
- Maintains class records
- Attends staff meetings as needed
- Attends continuing training as appropriate
- Notifies program director as soon as possible in case of absence
- Gives 2 weeks' notice if withdrawal becomes necessary before end of commitment
- Arranges for qualified, preapproved substitute in case of absence

Needed Qualifications

- Cheerful, positive attitude with people of all abilities
- Comfortable in and around water
- Has basic water-safety knowledge
- Is able to lead a class in an exercise routine confidently
- Is physically able to lead the class
- Has current CPR and first aid certification

Training and Job Preparation

- Attends orientation to program policy and class concept
- Works as an assistant leader for 4 weeks prior to leading a class
- Attends a monthly meeting

Supervision and Evaluation

- Program supervisor attends class and provides feedback on a monthly basis.
- Program supervisor is available to discuss questions, problems, or concerns.
- Formal evaluations and recommendations are available on request.

Minimum Time Commitment

6 months

Sample Goal Contracts

Appendix B

STARTER FITNESS CONTRACT*

Goals

I, ____, being of sound mind and body, do hereby proclaim that to the best of my ability I will

Signed ______________________

Witnessed ______________________

Date ______________________

I understand that my Starter Fitness Instructor and the YMCA Fitness Center Team are available for individual consultation to help me pursue a healthier lifestyle. I also understand that an integral component of wellness is self-responsibility and that my signature verifies my desire and commitment to accept the challenge of becoming the best that I can be.

---

*This form is reproduced with the permission of the YMCA of Metropolitan Milwaukee, Milwaukee, WI.

*Limited Warranty**

You are the owner of the most finely constructed, intricate and dependable device ever created—the human body.

Treat your body as you would any valuable precision instrument. Although ruggedly constructed to withstand the rigors of normal use, it may be damaged by lack of exercise, improper diet, smoking, and immoderate use of alcohol and other drugs.

Your body is warranted for 74 years to perform reliably the ordinary purposes for which it is intended. This warranty shall not apply to any body which has been subject to misuse, abuse, negligence, accident or failure to provide reasonable and necessary maintenance.

For example:

. . . if you smoke more than two packs of cigarettes a day, subtract eight years; between one and two packs a day, subtract six years; one-half to one pack a day, subtract three years.

. . . if you drink two cocktails a day, subtract one year; for each additional daily drink, subtract two years.

. . . for every ten pounds overweight, subtract one year.

. . . if you don't get much exercise at work, home, or play, subtract three years; if you do, add three years.

. . . if you are ambitious, aggressive, or nervous, subtract three years; if you have a relaxed approach to life, add three years.

. . . if you have an annual blood pressure check or are under treatment for the condition, add one year.

Owner's Obligation:

Proper care is necessary to obtain the maximum age limit. It is an obligation to periodically check to be certain your blood pressure is proper and your lifestyle in balance. A regular inspection is strongly recommended.

The undersigned understands the above conditions and limitations on the length of the warranty.

____

(Your Signature)

*This form is reproduced with the permission of the YMCA of Metropolitan Milwaukee, Milwaukee, WI.

Energy Expenditure in Household, Recreational, and Sports Activities (in kcal • min^{-1})

Appendix C

Activity	kcal•min^{-1}•kg^{-1}
Archery	0.065
Badminton	0.097
Bakery, general (F)	0.035
Basketball	0.138
Billiards	0.042
Bookbinding	0.038
Boxing	
in ring	0.222
sparring	0.138
Canoeing	
leisure	0.044
racing	0.103
Card playing	0.025
Carpentry, general	0.052
Carpet sweeping (F)	0.045
Carpet sweeping (M)	0.048
Circuit training	
Hydra-Fitness	0.132
Universal	0.116
Nautilus	0.092
Free Weights	0.086
Cleaning (F)	0.062
Cleaning (M)	0.058
Climbing hills	
with no load	0.121
with 5-kg load	0.129
with 10-kg load	0.140
with 20-kg load	0.147
Coal mining	
drilling coal, rock	0.094
erecting supports	0.088
shoveling coal	0.108
Cooking (F)	0.045
Cooking (M)	0.048
Cricket	
batting	0.083
bowling	0.090
Croquet	0.059
Cycling	
leisure, 5.5 mph	0.064
leisure, 9.4 mph	0.100
racing	0.169
Dancing	
Dancing (F)	
aerobic, medium	0.103
aerobic, intense	0.135
ballroom	0.051
choreographed	
"twist," "wiggle"	0.168
Digging trenches	0.145
Drawing (standing)	0.036
Eating (sitting)	0.023
Electrical work	0.058
Farming	
barn cleaning	0.135
driving harvester	0.040
driving tractor	0.037
feeding cattle	0.085
feeding animals	0.065
forking straw bales	0.138
milking by hand	0.054
milking by machine	0.023
shoveling grain	0.085
Field hockey	0.134
Fishing	0.062
Food shopping (F)	0.062
Food shopping (M)	0.058
Football	0.132
Forestry	
ax chopping, fast	0.297
ax chopping, slow	0.085
barking trees	0.123
carrying logs	0.186
felling trees	0.132
hoeing	0.091
planting by hand	0.109
sawing by hand	0.122
sawing, power	0.075

(Cont.)

Activity	$kcal \cdot min^{-1} \cdot kg^{-1}$
stacking firewood	0.088
trimming trees	0.129
weeding	0.072
Furriery	0.083
Gardening	
digging	0.126
hedging	0.077
mowing	0.112
raking	0.054
Golf	0.085
Gymnastics	0.066
Horse-grooming	0.128
Horse-racing	
galloping	0.137
trotting	0.110
walking	0.041
Ironing (F)	0.033
Ironing (M)	0.064
Judo	0.195
Jumping rope	
70 per min	0.162
80 per min	0.164
125 per min	0.177
145 per min	0.197
Knitting, sewing (F)	0.022
Knitting, sewing (M)	0.023
Locksmith	0.057
Lying at ease	0.022
Machine-tooling	
machining	0.048
operating lathe	0.052
operating punch press	0.088
tapping and drilling	0.065
welding	0.052
working sheet metal	0.048
Marching, rapid	0.142
Mopping floor (F)	0.062
Mopping floor (M)	0.058
Music playing	
accordion (sitting)	0.032
cello (sitting)	0.041
conducting	0.039
drums (sitting)	0.066
flute (sitting)	0.035
horn (sitting)	0.029
organ (sitting)	0.053
piano (sitting)	0.040
trumpet (standing)	0.031
violin (sitting)	0.045
woodwind (sitting)	0.032
Painting, inside	0.034
Painting, outside	0.077
Planting seedlings	0.070
Plastering	0.078
Printing	0.035
Racquetball	0.178
Running, cross-country	0.163
Running, horizontal	
11 min, 30 s per mile	0.135
9 min per mile	0.193
8 min per mile	0.208
7 min per mile	0.228
6 min per mile	0.252
5 min, 30 s per mile	0.289
Scraping paint	0.063
Scrubbing floors (F)	0.109
Scrubbing floors (M)	0.108
Shoe repair, general	0.045
Sitting quietly	0.021
Skiing, hard snow	
level, moderate speed	0.119
level, walking	0.143
uphill, maximum speed	0.274
Skiing, soft snow	
leisure (F)	0.111
leisure (M)	0.098
Skindiving, as frogman	
considerable motion	0.276
moderate motion	0.206
Snowshoeing, soft snow	0.166
Squash	0.212
Standing quietly (F)	0.025
Standing quietly (M)	0.027
Steel mill, working in	
fettling	0.089
forging	0.100
hand rolling	0.137
merchant mill rolling	0.145
removing slag	0.178
tending furnace	0.126
tipping molds	0.092
Stock clerking	0.054
Swimming	
back stroke	0.169
breast stroke	0.162
crawl, fast	0.156
crawl, slow	0.128
side stroke	0.122
treading, fast	0.170
treading, normal	0.062
Table tennis	0.068
Tailoring	
cutting	0.041
hand-sewing	0.032
machine-sewing	0.045
pressing	0.062
Tennis	0.109
Typing	
electric	0.027
manual	0.031
Volleyball	0.050
Walking, normal pace	
asphalt road	0.080
fields and hillsides	0.082
grass track	0.081
plowed field	0.077
Wallpapering	0.048
Watch repairing	0.025
Window cleaning (F)	0.059
Window cleaning (M)	0.058
Writing (sitting)	0.029

Note. Data from McArdle, W.D., Katch, F.I., and Katch, V.L.: Exercise Physiology. Lea & Febiger, Philadelphia, 1986. Data from E.W. Bannister and S.R. Brown, The relative energy requirements of physical activity in H.B. Falls, ed., Exercise Physiology, Academic Press, New York, 1968; E.T. Howley and M.E. Glover, The caloric costs of running and walking one mile for men and women, Medicine and Science in Sports 6:235, 1974. R. Passmore and J.V.G.A. Durnin, Human energy expenditure, Physiological Reviews, 35:801, 1955. Symbols (M) and (F) denote experiments for males and females, respectively.

Health Screening, Medical Clearance, and Informed-Consent Forms

Appendix D

The following five forms are taken from *Health Enhancement for America's Work Force—Program Guide* (YMCA of the USA, 1987). They can be reproduced and used as needed for your YMCA classes. The screening forms should be administered when participants enter a program and yearly thereafter. Copies of all completed participant forms should be retained in a records file for at least 3 years.

FORM I—HEALTH SCREEN FORM

Form I is the Health Screen Form. It obtains general information about the participant's physical condition. The form is completed by the participant to document information on age, height, weight, blood pressure, smoking, diabetes, heart problems, family history, and orthopedic and other problems. It also includes information on whom to contact in the event of an emergency. Form IA (Range of Recommended Body Weights) is used to determine the classification of current body weight (question 1). Individuals with heart or other problems that may limit exercise must obtain medical clearance from a physician before being allowed to participate in YMCA fitness testing or exercise programs.

FORM II—CARDIOVASCULAR DISEASE RISK FACTOR ESTIMATE

Form II provides a way to estimate the individual's risk for developing heart disease. It is completed and scored by the participant. (YMCA staff may have to help participants complete the items on blood pressure and heart rate.)

Form IA is again used to determine weight category (question 3). After staff have reviewed this form, it is used in an educational process to help participants evaluate some of their health habits and initiate steps to improve their lifestyles. Persons with high-risk scores (33 or greater) are required to obtain medical clearance from a physician before participating in fitness testing or exercise programs.

FORM III—MEDICAL CLEARANCE FORM

The Medical Clearance Form is used by the participant's physician to report any restrictions that should be placed on the participant during fitness testing or exercise programs. The physician should see both Form III and Form IIIA, which describe generally the YMCA fitness testing and exercise programs and the risks associated with each.

FORM IV—INFORMED CONSENT FOR FITNESS TESTING

The Informed Consent for Fitness Testing form insures that the participant is aware of the risks involved in the fitness testing procedures. It documents that a description of the testing procedures has been read and that all questions concerning those procedures have been answered satisfactorily.

FORM V—INFORMED CONSENT FOR EXERCISE PARTICIPATION

The Informed Consent for Exercise Participation form insures that the participant is aware of the risks involved in exercise. It documents that the description of the exercise program has been read and all questions concerning the exercise program have been answered to the participant's satisfaction.

WHEN AND HOW TO USE THE FORMS

The Health Screen Form (Form I) and the Cardiovascular Disease Risk Factor Estimate (Form II) should be completed before a participant starts any program, even if it is just an education class. The information obtained in Forms I and II is valuable for determining the level of a participant's health and cardiovascular risk. Note that Forms I and II are not intended to be medical exams but simply to obtain key health information.

Any person who responds affirmatively to questions 2, 5, 7, or 8 on the Health Screen Form or who scores 33 or higher on the Cardiovascular Disease Risk Factor Estimate may not participate in any fitness test or any exercise program until the Medical Clearance Form (Form III) is completed and signed by a physician.

The informed consent forms (Forms IV and V) are designed to notify participants of the inherent risks of fitness testing and exercise programs. Form IV (Informed Consent for Fitness Testing) should be given to any person registering for a fitness test. It should be read and signed before testing starts. Form V (Informed Consent for Exercise Participation) should be given to any participant in a supervised exercise program. It should be read and signed before exercise starts.

Form I—Health Screen Form

Name ______________________________ Date ______________________________

Male __________ Female __________ Age __________ Height __________ Weight __________

This form is intended to obtain relevant information about your health that will assist the staff in helping you with your program. Please answer all questions to the best of your knowledge.

1. Weight
   According to the attached recommended weight chart, is your current body weight
   ________ underweight? (more than 5 lb under ideal) ________ 5 to 19 lb overweight?
   ________ normal? (± 5 lb of ideal) ________ more than 20 lb overweight?
2. Blood Pressure
   Do you have high blood pressure? yes no
   Have you had high blood pressure in the past? yes no
   Are you on medication for high blood pressure? yes no
3. Smoking
   Do you smoke? yes no
   Are you a former smoker? yes no
   If yes, please give the date you quit. __________________________
4. Diabetes
   Do you have diabetes? yes no
5. Heart Problems
   Have you ever had a heart attack? yes no Heart surgery? yes no
   Angina? yes no
6. Family History
   Have any of your blood relatives had heart disease, heart surgery, or angina? yes no
7. Orthopedic Problems
   Do you have any serious orthopedic problems that would prevent you from exercising?
   yes no If yes, please explain.

   ____

   ____

   ____
8. Other Problems
   Do you have any reason to believe you should not exercise? yes no If yes, please explain.

   ____

   ____

   ____
9. Emergency
   Please list a relative whom we may contact in case of an emergency:

   Name ______________________________ Telephone ______________

   Relation ____

Form IA—Range of Recommended Body Weights Health Screen Form

Height	Weight in pounds	
	Men	Women
5'0"	—	96-125
5'1"	—	99-128
5'2"	112-141	102-131
5'3"	115-144	105-134
5'4"	118-148	108-138
5'5"	121-152	111-142
5'6"	124-156	114-146
5'7"	128-161	118-150
5'8"	132-166	122-154
5'9"	136-170	126-158
5'10"	140-174	130-163
5'11"	144-179	134-168
6'0"	148-184	138-173
6'1"	152-189	—
6'2"	156-194	—
6'3"	160-199	—
6'4"	164-204	—

Note. From *Implementing Health/Fitness Programs* (p. 111) by R.W. Patton, J.M. Corry, L.R. Gettman, and J.S. Graf, 1986, Champaign, IL: Human Kinetics. Copyright 1986 by R.W. Patton, J.M. Corry, L.R. Gettman, and J.S. Graf. Adapted by permission.

Form II—Cardiovascular Disease Risk Factor Estimate

Name ______________________________

						Date			
1. Age	10-20 Years 1	21-30 Years 2	31-40 Years 3	41-50 years 4	51-60 years 6	> 60 years 8			
2. Heredity: parents and siblings	No family history of CVD 1	One with CVD over 60 years 2	Two with CVD over 60 years 3	One death from CVD under 60 years 4	Two deaths from CVD under 60 years 6	Three deaths from CVD under 60 years 7			
3. Weight: refer to Form IA	More than 5 lbs. below standard weight 0	−5 to +5 lbs. of standard weight 1	5 to 20 lbs overweight 2	21 to 35 lbs overweight 3	36-50 lbs overweight 5	51-65 lbs overweight 7			
4. Tobacco smoking	Nonuser 0	Occasional cigar or pipe 1	Cigarettes 10 or less/day 2	Cigarettes 11-20 per day 4	Cigarettes 21-30 per day 6	Cigarettes over 30/ day 10			
5. Exercise	Intensive job and recreational exertion 0	Moderate job and recreational exertion 1	Sedentary job and intensive recreation 2	Sedentary job and moderate recreation 4	Sedentary job and light recreation 6	Sedentary job. No special exercise 8			
6. Cholesterol and triglycerides	Low-fat diet. No sugar intake 0	Below-average fat and sugar intake 2	Normal fat and sugar intake 3	High-fat and normal sugar intake 5	High fat and sugar intake 6	Excessive fat and sugar intake 10			
7. Systolic blood pressure	< 111 mmHg 0	111-130 mmHg 1	131-140 mmHg 2	141-160 mmHg 3	161-180 mmHg 5	Above 180 mmHg 7			
8. Diastolic blood pressure	< 80 mmHg 0	80-85 mmHg 1	86-90 mmHg 2	91-95 mmHg 4	96-100 mmHg 7	Above 100 mmHg 9			
9. Gender	Female < 40 years 1	Female 40-50 years 2	Female > 50 years 4	Male 5	Male (paunchy) 6	Male (obese) 7			
10. Resting heart rate Men / Women	< 56 / < 65 1	57-64 / 66-70 2	65-70 / 71-75 3	71-77 / 76-82 4	78-81 / 83-86 5	> 82 / > 87 7			
11. Stress	No stress 1	Occasional mild stress 2	Frequent mild stress 3	Frequent moderate stress 4	Frequent high stress 5	Constant high stress 7			
12. Present CVD symptoms	None 0	Occasional fast pulse and/or irregular rhythm 2	Frequent fast pulse and/or irregular rhythm 4	Occasional angina 6	Exertional angina 8	Frequent angina (exertional and resting) 10			
13. Past personal CVD history	Completely benign 0	CVD symptoms not MD confirmed 2	CVD mild MD confirmed BP medication 4	CVD moderate. Occasional symptoms 6	CVD severe frequent symptoms 8	Hospitalized for CVD 10			
14. Diabetes	No symptoms. Negative family history 0	Latent positive family history 1	Elevated blood glucose 3	Mild dietary control 5	Moderate oral medication control 7	Severe insulin control 9			
15. Gout	No symptoms. Negative family history 0	Family history 1	Elevated uric acid (>8 mg/dl) no symptoms 2	New onset Gout. Medication control 3	Repeated chronic gouty attacks 5	Gout with renal and osteo complications 8			
						TOTAL SCORE			

If you score:

6-14 = Risk well below average
15-19 = Risk below average
20-25 = Risk generally average
26-32 = Risk moderate
33-40 = Risk dangerous; you must reduce your score
41-55 = Risk very dangerous; you must reduce your score immediately
56 + = Risk extreme; urgent medical treatment recommended

Remarks: ______________________________

____

____

____

Note. Adapted by permission of the New York State Education Department's HEALTHY STATE PROGRAM, Albany, N.Y.

Form III—Medical Clearance Form

Dear Doctor:

______________________________ has applied for enrollment in the fitness testing and/or
name of applicant

exercise programs at the YMCA. The fitness testing program involves a submaximal test for cardiorespiratory fitness, body composition analysis, flexibility test, and muscular strength and endurance tests. The exercise programs are designed to start easy and become progressively more difficult over a period of time. A more detailed description of the testing and exercise programs is attached in Form IIIA. All fitness tests and exercise programs will be administered by qualified personnel trained in conducting exercise tests and exercise programs.

By completing the form below, however, you are not assuming any responsibility for our administration of the fitness testing and/or exercise programs. If you know of any medical or other reasons why participation in the fitness testing and/or exercise programs by the applicant would be unwise, please indicate so on this form.

If you have any questions about the YMCA fitness testing and/or exercise programs, please call.

Report of Physician

___ I know of no reason why the applicant may not participate.

___ I believe the applicant can participate, but I urge caution because

____

____

___ The applicant should not engage in the following activities:

____

____

___ I recommend that the applicant NOT participate.

Physician signature ______________________________ Date ______________

Address ______________________________ Telephone ______________

City and State ______________________________ Zip ______________

Form IIIA—Description of Fitness Testing and Exercise Programs

Dear Doctor:

The YMCA fitness testing and/or exercise programs for which the participant has applied are described as follows:

Fitness testing—The purpose of the fitness testing program is to evaluate cardiorespiratory fitness, body composition, flexibility, and muscular strength and endurance. The cardiorespiratory fitness test involves a submaximal test that may include a bench step test, a cycle ergometer test, or a one-mile walk for best time test. Body composition is analyzed by taking several skinfold measures to calculate percentage of body fat. Flexibility is determined by the sit-and-reach test. Muscular strength may be determined by an upper-body bench press test or a lower-body leg extension test. Muscular endurance may be evaluated by the one-minute, bent-knee sit-up test or the endurance bench press test.

Exercise programs—The purpose of the exercise programs is to develop and maintain cardiorespiratory fitness, body composition, flexibility, and muscular strength and endurance. A specific exercise plan will be given to the participant based on needs and interests and your recommendations. All exercise programs include warm-up, exercise at target heart rate, and cool-down (except for muscular strength and endurance training, in which target heart rate is not a factor). The programs may involve walking, jogging, swimming, or cycling (outdoor and stationary); participation in exercise fitness, rhythmic aerobic exercise, or choreographed fitness classes; or calisthenics or strength training. All programs are designed to place a gradually increasing workload on the body in order to improve overall fitness and muscular strength. The rate of progression is regulated by exercise target heart rate and/or perceived effort of exercise.

In both the fitness testing and exercise programs, the reaction of the cardiorespiratory system cannot be predicted with complete accuracy. There is a risk of certain changes that might occur during or following exercise. These changes might include abnormalities of blood pressure and/or heart rate. YMCA exercise instructors are certified in CPR, and emergency procedures are posted in the exercise facility.

In addition to your medical approval and recommendations, the participant will be asked to sign informed consent forms that explain the risks of fitness testing and exercise participation before the programs are initiated.

Form IV—Informed Consent for Fitness Testing

Name ____
(please print)

The purpose of the fitness testing program is to evaluate cardiorespiratory fitness, body composition, flexibility, and muscular strength and endurance. The cardiorespiratory fitness test involves a submaximal test that may include a bench step test, a cycle ergometer test, or a one-mile walk test. Body composition is analyzed by taking several skinfold measures to calculate percentage of body fat. Flexibility is determined by the sit-and-reach test. Muscular strength may be determined by an upper-body bench press test or a lower-body leg extension test. Muscular endurance may be evaluated by the one-minute, bent-knee sit-up test or the endurance bench press test.

I understand that I am responsible for monitoring my own condition throughout the tests, and should any unusual symptoms occur, I will cease my participation and inform the instructor of the symptoms.

In signing this consent form, I affirm that I have read this form in its entirety and that I understand the description of the tests and their components. I also affirm that my questions regarding the fitness testing program have been answered to my satisfaction.

In the event that a medical clearance must be obtained prior to my participation in the fitness testing program, I agree to consult my physician and obtain written permission from my physician prior to the commencement of any fitness tests.

Also, in consideration for being allowed to participate in the fitness testing program, I agree to assume the risk of such testing, and further agree to hold harmless the YMCA and its staff members conducting such testing from any and all claims, suits, losses, or related causes of action for damages, including, but not limited to, such claims that may result from my injury or death, accidental or otherwise, during, or arising in any way from, the testing program.

____ ____________________
(Signature of participant) (Date)

____ ____________________
(Person administering tests) (Date)

Form V—Informed Consent for Exercise Participation

I desire to engage voluntarily in the YMCA exercise program in order to attempt to improve my physical fitness. I understand that the activities are designed to place a gradually increasing workload on the cardiorespiratory system and to thereby attempt to improve its function. The reaction of the cardiorespiratory system to such activities can't be predicted with complete accuracy. There is a risk of certain changes that might occur during or following the exercise. These changes might include abnormalities of blood pressure or heart rate.

I understand that the purpose of the exercise program is to develop and maintain cardiorespiratory fitness, body composition, flexibility, and muscular strength and endurance. A specific exercise plan will be given to me, based on my needs and interests and my doctor's recommendations. All exercise programs include warm-up, exercise at target heart rate, and cool-down. The programs may involve walking, jogging, swimming, or cycling (outdoor and stationary); participation in exercise fitness, rhythmic aerobic exercise, or choreographed fitness classes; or calisthenics or strength training. All programs are designed to place a gradually increasing workload on the body in order to improve overall fitness. The rate of progression is regulated by exercise target heart rate and perceived effort of exercise.

I understand that I am responsible for monitoring my own condition throughout the exercise program and should any unusual symptoms occur, I will cease my participation and inform the instructor of the symptoms.

In signing this consent form, I affirm that I have read this form in its entirety and that I understand the nature of the exercise program. I also affirm that my questions regarding the exercise program have been answered to my satisfaction.

In the event that a medical clearance must be obtained prior to my participation in the exercise program, I agree to consult my physician and obtain written permission from my physician prior to the commencement of any exercise program.

Also, in consideration for being allowed to participate in the YMCA exercise program, I agree to assume the risk of such exercise, and further agree to hold harmless the YMCA and its staff members conducting the exercise program from any and all claims, suits, losses, or related causes of action for damages, including, but not limited to, such claims that may result from my injury or death, accidental or otherwise, during, or arising in any way from, the exercise program.

____ ______________

(Signature of participant) (Date)

Please print:

Name ______________________________ Date of birth ______________

Address ____

Street City State Zip

Telephone ____

Name of personal physician ______________________________

Physician's address ______________________________________

Physician's phone ______________________________________

Limitations and medications ______________________________

References

American College of Sports Medicine. (1986). *Guidelines for exercise testing and prescription* (3rd ed.). Philadelphia: Lea & Febiger.

American Heart Association. (1972). *Exercise testing and training of apparently healthy individuals: A handbook for physicians*. New York: Author.

American Heart Association. (1975). *Exercise testing and training of individuals with heart disease or at high risk for its development: A handbook for physicians*. New York: Author.

Åstrand, P.-O., & Rhyming, I. (1954). A nomogram for calculation of aerobic capacity (physical fitness) from pulse rate during submaximal work. *Journal of Applied Physiology*, **7**, 218-221.

Brozek, J., Grande, F., Anderson, J.T., & Keys, A. (1963). Densitometric analysis of body composition: Revision of some quantitative assumptions. *Annals of the New York Academy of Science*, **110**, 113.

Cureton, T.K., Jr. (1941). Flexibility as an aspect of physical fitness. *Research Quarterly Supplement*, **12**, 388-390.

Golding, L.A. (1988). *Differences in skinfold measurements using different calipers*. Unpublished manuscript.

Gruber, J.S., & Pollock, M.L. (1988). *Comparison of Harpenden and Lange calipers in predicting body composition*. Unpublished manuscript.

Jackson, A.S., & Pollock, M.L. (1978). Generalized equations for predicting body density of man. *British Journal of Nutrition*, **40**, 497-504.

Johnson, B.L., & Nelson, J.K. (1979). *Practical measurement for evaluation in physical education*. Minneapolis: Burgess.

McArdle, W.D., Katch, F.I., & Katch, V.L. (1981). *Exercise physiology*. Philadelphia: Lea & Febiger.

Scott, M.G., & French, E. (1959). *Measurement and evaluation in physical education*. Dubuque, IA: Brown.

Siri, W.E. (1956). Gross composition of the body. In J.H. Lawrence & C.A. Tobias (Eds.), *Advances in biological and medical physics* (Vol. 4) (pp. 239-280). New York: Academic Press.

Sjostrand, T. (1947). Changes in the respiratory organs of workmen at an ore melting works. *Acta Medica Scandinavica*, **128** (Suppl. 196), 687-699.

Wilmore, J.H. (1983). Body composition in sport and exercise: Directions for future research. *Medicine and Science in Sports and Exercise*, **15**, 21.

YMCA of the USA. (1987). *Health enhancement for America's work force—Program guide*. Champaign, IL: Human Kinetics.

Index

Page numbers in italics refer to figures.

Y's Way to Stress Management Leader's Guide, 7, 164